A History of the Council for the Education and Training of Health Visitors

*An Account of its Establishment and Field of Activities
1962–1975*

ELAINE WILKIE

London
GEORGE ALLEN & UNWIN
Boston   Sydney

First published in 1979

GEORGE ALLEN & UNWIN LTD
40 Museum Street, London WC1A 1LU

© Council for the Education and Training of
Health Visitors, 1979

British Library Cataloguing in Publication Data

Wilkie, Elaine
    A history of the Council for the Education and
Training of Health Visitors.
    1. Great Britain. Council for the Education and
Training of Health Visitors – History
    I. Title
362.1'4'071141   RT81.G7   78–40855

ISBN 0–04–610011–3

Typeset in 11 on 13 point Baskerville by Trade Linotype
and printed in Great Britain
by Unwin Brothers Limited, Old Woking, Surrey

A HISTORY OF THE COUNCIL FOR THE EDUCATION AND TRAINING OF HEALTH VISITORS

Also published by the Council for the Education
and Training of Health Visitors.

*The Work of the Nursing Team in General
Practice.*
*An Investigation into the Principles of Health
Visiting.*

We cannot dissociate ourselves from our inheritance. Our problem is to continue an evolutionary process; to gather a sense of inspiration, endurance and settlement from the ancient ways and to direct them in new paths.

SIR GEORGE NEWMAN

1923

Introduction by the Chairman of the Council for the Education and Training of Health Visitors

All who were concerned with the first years of the Council's existence will know how much is owed to the author of this book, Miss Elaine Wilkie, and while she alone is able to write this intimate account of the remarkable developments which took place during these years, her natural modesty precludes adequate reference in the text to the part she herself played.

To change the health visitors' courses from the fragmentary state of earlier years and to establish them as well-respected developments in university and polytechnic departments and in colleges of further education was no mean task. To this was added an increase in student places by $2\frac{1}{2}$ times, the refinement of a newly-designed syllabus and the requirement for both health visitor tutor and fieldwork teacher courses.

This book gives an account of the stages in these developments and why some ideas came to fruition and others did not. To this fascinating history are added glimpses into the minds of those involved and the external and internal influences prevailing at the time.

Those of us who follow on, as well as others interested in the development of education for a profession, will find this account both readable and illuminating. In spite of the modest style of writing we can be left in no doubt about the courage and vision of those pioneers, both those within the Council and those involved in the service and in teaching, who pressed ahead in laying the sound educational foundation on which health visitor education and training is now built.

CLIFFORD BUTLER

Foreword

The Council for the Education and Training of Health Visitors was established in 1962 and is, therefore, with the exception of the Northern Ireland Council for Nurses and Midwives, the latest of the statutory bodies concerned with nursing. Its constitution and powers differ from those of its sister councils as do the resources upon which it draws for the institution and regulation of training. It adopts a different approach both to the establishment of a training programme and to the maintenance of standards. This is an account of its work between 1962 and 1975.

So many people have helped in the making of this record that it is difficult to name them all, but mention must be made of some without whose interest and assistance this account could not have been written. I will begin with the hero of the story, the Council. Its Director Miss Batley gave constant encouragement and ensured that the necessary resources for the collection of data might be available; the professional staff willingly retrieved information for me on their own specialities. In particular I must mention Miss Tarbuck who acted as the essential link between an author, on occasion 500 miles further north, and the headquarters with its central record system.

The Royal College of Nursing, the Health Visitors' Association and the Standing Conference of Health Visitor Training Centres kindly gave me access to committee papers relating to the establishment of the Council, and the Scottish Home and Health Department assisted me in the recall of certain work carried out by the Scottish Advisory Committee in its early years.

This account will be used as the basis for further study and I am greatly indebted to Miss Hockey, Director of the Nursing Studies Research Unit at Edinburgh University, for much support and helpful advice, and to those members of the present or former Councils, Mrs M. Klinger, Dr P. E. O'Connell and Professor I. M. Richardson, who read and commented on a draft.

I should like to express my appreciation to George Allen & Unwin Ltd. for their assistance in publishing this book.

It is expected that following a recommendation of the Committee on Nursing a new Central Council will be established incorporating all the existing statutory bodies and that this will mean the disappearance of this Council in its present form. It is hoped that some of the lessons learned over the twelve years by this singular and lively institution may be of interest to those concerned in the foundation of the new organisation as well as to the many health visitors who welcomed and supported 'their' Council in the intervening years.

Abbreviations

Council or Health Visitor Council refers to the Council for the Education and Training of Health Visitors (CTHV before 1971, CETHV after 1971).

Social Work Council refers to the Central Council for Education and Training in Social Work.

CTSW (until 1971)	Council for Training in Social Work.
CCETSW (after 1971)	Central Council for Education and Training in Social Work.
DHSS	Department of Health and Social Security.
SHHD	Scottish Home and Health Department.
HVA	Health Visitors' Association.
SHVA	Scottish Health Visitors' Association.
Rcn	Royal College of Nursing.
HC	Proceedings in Parliament – House of Commons.
HL	Proceedings in Parliament – House of Lords.

Contents

system by The National Foundation for Educational Research; Fieldwork: the range of experience.

Chapter 1

INTRODUCTION

Begin at the beginning and go on to
the end then stop.
Alice through the Looking Glass—
LEWIS CARROLL

The only problem in following the excellent advice given by the
Red King to Alice is to find a beginning and an end. In the
case of the Council, the basis for its life was laid before 1962 and,
as yet at least, its existence has not been terminated. While this
publication therefore concentrates on the years 1962 until 1975,
i.e. from the inauguration of the Council to the separation of
resources from those of the Central Council for Education and
Training in Social Work, the sister organisation with which it
shares the Health Visiting and Social Work (Training) Act 1962,
it will include some account of earlier events in order to give an
understanding both of the scope and limitations. It will be necessary
to refer briefly, first, to the pressure exerted by the professional
groups of health visitors for inquiry into areas of work and training, second to comment on the reports of two Working Parties
established under the Chairmanship of Sir Wilson Jameson[1] and
Dame Eileen Younghusband[2] respectively, and third to reactions
to the subsequent Act.

A fuller list of the many developments which have relevance to
the establishment of the health visiting service, its training and
subsequent development appears in Appendix 1.

The functions of the new Council, i.e. the Council for the
Training of Health Visitors offered some interesting contrasts with
those of the other statutory bodies concerned with nursing. Its
powers were set out in Section 2 of the Act.

2 (1) The Council for the Training of Health Visitors—

    (a) shall promote the training of health visitors by seeking to secure suitable facilities for the training of persons intending to become health visitors by approving such courses as suitable to be attended by such persons and by seeking to attract persons to such courses;

    (b) if it appears to them that adequate provision is not being made for the further training of health visitors, shall provide or secure the provision of courses for this purpose;

    (c) may conduct or make arrangements for the conduct of examinations in connection with such courses as are mentioned in the preceding paragraphs; and

    (d) may carry out or assist other persons in carrying out research into matters relevant to the training of health visitors.

  (2) An approval under paragraph (a) of subsection (1) of this section shall be given by the Council in accordance with rules made by the Council and approved by the Health Ministers, and those rules may specify subjects to be comprised in the courses to be approved and shall specify the conditions for admission to the courses and for the award by the Council of certificates of their successful completion.

STATUTORY BODIES BEFORE 1962

Prior to the Act, in common with nursing and midwifery training, separate institutions were responsible for health visitor training in England and Scotland; Wales, where there was one training school, was included in the English system as was Northern Ireland where training was introduced in 1948. In contrast to nursing for which General Nursing Councils had been established for Wales and England and for Scotland in 1919, the responsibility for establishing and maintaining standards, laying down a syllabus and conducting examinations was that of two organisations, the Royal Society of Health in England and the Royal Sanitary Association of Scotland. These had diverse functions which included regulative elements for certain workers such as health visitors, nursery nurses and public health inspectors. Training and Examination Committees advised the respective Councils on the nature of syllabus and examination and prepared recommendations on training schools for the Government Departments concerned. Although as a result of representations from such bodies as the Standing Conference of Health Visitor Training Centres, the health visitor membership of the committee had increased in the post-war years, few health visitors became members of the Councils of the statutory bodies and there were no health visitor members of staff. Considerable changes had been effected in the examination syllabus in both England and Scotland but this was not matched by a change in the choice of examiners. The list was still composed exclusively of medical officers, maternity and child health officers, and health visitors. It tended to reflect an earlier concentration on the environmental aspects of health which had been overtaken in many instances by a widening of the curriculum in training schools. Something of a discrepancy between the material taught and the subjects of the examination was, therefore, developing. Many other factors contributed to a growing realisation that the pre-war pattern did not meet contemporary needs and pressure mounted from professional and training bodies for an investigation of the role of the health visitor and therefore the appropriate training. The Working Parties created, for health visitors in 1953 and for social workers in 1955, reported in 1956[1] and 1959[2] respectively.

PROPOSED RELATIONSHIP WITH THE SOCIAL WORK COUNCIL

There had always been a shadowy area of responsibility in the work of health visitor and social worker and a possible area of overlap. Over the years this has been the cause of debate and, on occasion, dispute concerning their respective roles, and the proposal in the Health Visitor and Social Work Training Bill that the training of the two workers might be related by the formation of two Councils with a common Chairman, and some members in common, was not greeted with marked enthusiasm.

An inquiry by the Health Visitors' Association (then named the Women Public Health Officers' Association) showed that of their thirty-four centres, twenty-three would have preferred a completely autonomous body to be responsible for health visitors.[3] The Royal College of Nursing, Public Health Section, would initially have welcomed some closer relationship with the General Nursing Council[4] but when the Rcn and HVA joined for discussion they agreed that sharing with the Social Work Council might be more appropriate. There was, however, much concern over the appointment of the common Chairman and this matter was raised in debate by Mr Kenneth Robinson.[5] There was also considerable dispute over the nature of the membership. The professional bodies feared too much emphasis on employers' interests and too little on professional interests, a matter which was also raised in the course of the Parliamentary debates.

THE STANDING CONFERENCE OF HEALTH VISITOR TRAINING CENTRES

In addition to the two professional organisations concerned with health visitors, a strong pressure group existed in the Standing Conference of Health Visitor Training Centres. This body, which grew from the Joint Consultative Council of Health Visitor Training Centres, was given its new name and a slightly different membership in September 1945 and had then the following remit:

1. To appoint eight representatives of training centres to the Health Visitor Examination Committee of the Royal Sanitary Institute.[6]
2. To consider questions related to recruitment and selection of candidates for training.
3. To consider from time to time, questions relating to training of health visitors (other than matters dealt with by the Health Visitor Examination Committee with the agreement of the appointed members of Standing Conference on that Committee), and to make recommendations to the Minister on any such matters on which he may seek their advice or on which they wish to offer representations.

Membership consisted of two delegates from each training centre; a chairman and other honorary officers were elected from among the members. Finance was obtained from affiliation fees paid by each centre and the first meeting was held on 24 January 1946.

In the years since its inception, the Standing Conference has been able to exercise much influence on a number of improvements, for example, the widening of the Panel of Examiners to include non-medical representatives, in 1952, and comment on such matters as class size, 'schools with less than twelve students are uneconomic and should link with others for example with social science courses'. The Standing Conference also commented on the lack of outside lecturers in some schools, inadequate expenditure on libraries and the lack of promotion prospects in the independent centres, i.e. not Local Health Authority, Local Education Authority or university directed schools.

The Standing Conference commented on the Jameson Report, drawing attention to the failure to clarify the position of the tutor and particularly her training. This body by its very nature therefore obviously would be one of those most closely affected by the proposals for a new Council. Its members expressed themselves as 'very unhappy about the relationship with the Social Work Council' and pressed strongly for an independent chairman.[7] In the view of the Conference, the Health Visitor Certificate could not be equated with the certificate to be set up for social workers since the former was a second professional qualification obtained after general nurse training and state registration.

After this lapse of time it is difficult to determine the underlying philosophy which led to the linking of the two bodies. Certainly in the debates in the House of Lords the Bill was introduced for its second reading as being designed to 'forge a link' between two workers who would of necessity be serving the community in very close contact.[8] The possibility of creating a completely new kind of worker had been raised on a number of occasions, e.g. a paper by Fraser Brockington and I. G. Davis.[9] Alternatively this may merely have been an administrative convenience. The results, however, of putting the two Councils together have probably not been those either foreseen or hoped for by the originators of the bill.

IMPLICATIONS OF THE NEW COUNCIL'S CONSTITUTION

A brief exposition of the Council's life is not the place to attempt to evaluate the many factors which influenced policy and the ways in which it has developed. In preparing evidence for the Committee on Nursing[10] the Council drew attention to a number of these. Stress should be laid, however, on certain novel features in the composition of the Council. It differed from that of other training bodies in nursing, one of the most important features being the appointment of a chairman who did not belong to either the social work or health visitor profession. While this was a matter of great concern to health visitors who had hoped for a chairman selected from among their own number, there was obvious advantage in a situation in which there was to be some sharing of resources with another group or profession in having a common chairman. Such an appointment could bring the subtle benefit of an objective view in debate where too often argument could be distorted by a lack of diverse opinion. The Council members were appointed following consultation as outlined in the first schedule to the Act:

Status and Composition[11]
1. The Council for the Training of Health Visitors shall consist of a chairman and thirty-one other members and the Council for Training in Social Work of a chairman and thirty-two other members, and each of those Councils shall be a body corporate.
2. The Privy Council shall appoint one person to be chairman of both Councils.
3. The other members of the Council for the Training of Health Visitors shall be appointed as follows:
   (a) fourteen by the Health Ministers;
   (b) six by the Health Ministers and the Minister of Education;
   (c) three by the County Councils' Association;
   (d) one by the London County Council;
   (e) three by the Association of Municipal Corporations;

(f) one by the Association of County Councils in Scotland;

(g) one by the Convention of Royal Burghs of Scotland;

(h) one by the Scottish Counties of Cities Association;

(i) one by the Governor of Northern Ireland.

4. Refers to the membership of the Council for Training in Social Work.

5. Of the members mentioned in sub-paragraph (a) of paragraph 3 of this Schedule thirteen shall be appointed as follows :

(a) eight after consultation with associations appearing to the Health Ministers to represent health visitors;

(b) three after consultation with the British Medical Association and the Society of Medical Officers of Health;

(c) two after consultation with the General Nursing Council for England and Wales and the General Nursing Council for Scotland.

6. The members mentioned in sub-paragraph (b) of paragraph 3 of this Schedule shall be appointed after consultation with such universities and other bodies concerned with the training of health visitors as the Health Ministers and the Minister of Education think fit.

7 and 8 Refer to the membership of the Council for Training in Social Work.

9. In making any appointments under this Schedule regard shall be had to the desirability of securing an association between the two Councils and, in particular, the County Councils' Association and the Association of Municipal Corporations shall each appoint one person as a member of both Councils.

10. Of the members of each Council who are appointed by the Health Ministers, one, at least, shall be a fully registered medical practitioner engaged in general medical practice, and that member shall be among those appointed after consultation with the British Medical Association and the Society of Medical Officers of Health.

11. The Health Ministers and the Minister of Education shall ensure that one member at least of each Council is a person

who at the time of his appointment is ordinarily resident in Wales and shall, if necessary, make their appointments accordingly.

The system was intended to provide for an even geographical distribution of membership. In its turn this could develop an understanding of the varying patterns of work which a health visitor might encounter in the United Kingdom and the implications of this for the design of training. Although the link with the Social Work Council had a cool reception from the health visitors, the fact that it, unlike the Health Visitor Council, did not have predecessors may have been responsible for the greater flexibility given to both bodies. This was not an unmixed blessing: the Health Visitor Training Council had great autonomy in that it did not have to seek formal approval of a Central Government Department before establishing training but equally it had no powers in relation to the practice of the health visitor and consequently to the quality of experience available to students. Here a distinction may be drawn between the health visitor operating in a statutorily required service[12] with a certificate required by regulation[13] (in England and Wales at that time) and the social worker operating in a service without such well-defined boundaries and, by very reason of the lack of definition, able to approach training, untrammelled by the rigidity of long established practice.

When the two Councils took office in 1962, each was to have a small professional staff and a shared secretariat. In effect this meant that advice on policy and administration came from a triad, i.e. a Joint Secretary and two Chief Professional Advisers. Close co-operation and consultation among the three would be an essential element in the success of the new venture.

The inauguration of both Councils took place on 25 October 1962 at Caxton Hall in London; the inaugural address being given to both Councils by Lord Newton, Joint Parliamentary Secretary to the Minister of Health.

REFERENCES

1 *An Inquiry into Health Visiting* (Jameson Report), HMSO 1956.
2 *Report of the Working Party on Social Workers in the Local Authority Health and Welfare Services* (Younghusband Report), HMSO 1959.
3 *Women Public Health Officers Proceedings of Committees*, 1962.
4 *Royal College of Nursing Proceedings of Public Health Central Sectional Committees*, 1961.
5 HC Debate (1961–62) 665, c.1692.
6 The Royal Sanitary Institute was founded in 1876 and was renamed in 1955 'The Royal Society for the Promotion of Health', now commonly known as 'The Royal Society of Health'.
7 Standing Conference of Health Visitor Training Centres, *Proceedings of Conference,* 9.12.60.
8 HL Debate (1961–62) 240, c.1123.
9 Brockington, F. and Davis, I. G. 'The Need for a Revision in the Training of the Health Visitor'. *Public Health*, April 1949.
10 CTHV *Evidence to the Committee on Nursing*, 1970.
11 The Health Visiting and Social Work (Training Act), 1962, has been amended by:
   1. The Local Authority Social Service Act 1970, Section II, renaming CTHV and CTSW. This was brought about in the UK on 1 October 1971 by SI 1971. No. 1221 (C.31).
   2. SI 1971. No. 1241 relating to CCETSW.
   3. The NHS Reorganisation Act 1973, page 83, paragraph 102 which amended (3).
12 The National Health Service Act 1946, Section 24.
13 The National Health Service (Qualifications of Health Visitors and Tuberculosis Visitors) SI 1948. No. 1415.

Chapter 2

SETTING ABOUT THE TASK

I had three encouragements. 1. A smooth calm sea.
2. The tide rising and setting in to the shore. 3. What
little wind there was blew one towards the land . . .
I found two saws, an axe and a hammer and with this
cargo I put to sea.

Robinson Crusoe—DANIEL DEFOE

TASKS AWAITING THE NEW COUNCIL

The delay of over six years in the implementation of the Jameson
Report,[1] itself the result of pressure sustained over an even longer
period, produced a zeal for building a new and effective training
which might well be equalled by Robinson Crusoe's determination
to build his shelter and make use of the resources at his disposal. In
his opening remarks at the first meeting of the Health Visitor
Council, the Chairman, Sir John Wolfenden, outlined five areas
to which the Council should direct its attention urgently.[2] These
were :

(a) A revision of the syllabus for training for health visitors.
(b) A consideration of the part played by the Royal Society
of Health and the Royal Sanitary Association of Scotland
in the examination of the health visitor.
(c) A consideration of the supervision of students in practical
work.
(d) Discussion to consider the best pattern of relationships to
establish with the Standing Conference of Representatives
of Health Visitor Training Centres.

(e) Consideration must be given to improving recruitment of students to training courses and to the best means of obtaining candidates of the best quality.

Two panels were immediately established, one to consider syllabus and examination procedure and the other to consider fieldwork training. No steps were taken at the first meeting to pursue the problems involved in recruitment.

The diverse group forming the membership of this Council (see Appendix II) could be expected to take some time to form a coherent whole. Some members were experienced as elected representatives in Local Government: some had not had previous experience of nurse or health visitor training, but were well versed in the mainstream of education. Some of the medical officer members had extensive experience in the community service, but their relationship to the health visitor was within a hierarchical system which did not necessarily give an understanding of the aims and aspirations of this particular group of nurses. Meanwhile the health visitors were only too well aware of the many shortcomings in their service and its training and were anxious to attack these with vigour. The Council encountered a variety of problems in its first year, many the inevitable accompaniment of the establishment of a totally new organisation. The Ministry of Health provided accommodation for meetings and also provided administrative and secretarial support in the absence of a joint secretary. This absence of an identifiable base was significant in the speed, or otherwise, with which the Council was able to begin its work. It also affected the development in these early months of a sense of common purpose in the total membership of the Council. The Chief Professional Adviser, although appointed in December 1962, was on the staff of the University of Manchester with a continuing responsibility to students until the end of the academic year, i.e. 1962–63. A system of commuting between the two cities had to be developed although a base in London from April 1963 was provided for her and her colleague on the Social Work Council at the Ministry of Health. By July 1963 the first Joint Secretary Mr H. Croly CBE, had been appointed and premises found. These, however, required considerable adaptation and if Robinson

Crusoe's saw, axe and hammer were not required, the new Secretary found a screwdriver indispensable in the assembly of some of the equipment. The Council was not able to hold a meeting in its own home until July 1964. This was in Clifton House, in the centre of London, where the Council is still based.

CHAIRMANSHIP OF THE COUNCIL

An important event was the change in chairmanship in the first year. Sir John Wolfenden was appointed Chairman of the University Grants Committee and announced at the Council meeting on 25 June that it would be necessary for him to resign. The demands that the new office would make upon his time could not be reconciled with those of the two new and developing Councils. Much of the acceptance of the concept of two Councils with shared resources had been due to the respect held for Sir John Wolfenden and although his term of office was brief, his determination and energy enabled the Councils to get underway with their extensive tasks. In a very practical sense, he was able to ensure that they found a suitable base in central London and established their separate existence from that of the Government Departments. Sir John Wolfenden was able to announce the appointment of Sir Charles Morris KCMG, later Lord Morris of Grasmere, whom he introduced to the Council at the June (1963) meeting.

The appointment of the Secretary, the provision of temporary accommodation, first at Alexander Fleming House and later in Knightsbridge, and the organisation of a supporting staff, released professional staff to devote thought and energy to visiting existing training schools in order to prepare material for the panels and to begin the establishment of contact with related organisations.

Reference has already been made to the composition of the Council. It took some time for the members to accept a different way of working to that of other professional organisations or to the previous training bodies. Members had to consider the nature of their relationship towards supporting Government Departments. Some were particularly resistant to the fact that certain panels had been appointed in advance of the first Council meeting and that the pattern of suggesting the format of panels from the Chair continued. Health visitor members were especially anxious to exercise their new found responsibility in relation to training.

ESTABLISHMENT AND ROLE OF THE NATIONAL COMMITTEES

There is a further aspect of the development of a uniform policy which is too important to leave to a later stage in this account. Reference has already been made to the somewhat muted welcome given to the proposed Council in 1961–62. The fact that it would serve all the countries in the United Kingdom was not immediately acceptable to everyone. The Scottish health visitors, accustomed to the existence of a separate examination body, i.e. The Royal Sanitary Association of Scotland as well as the Scottish General Nursing Council and Central Midwives' Board for Scotland, had hoped to have their own organisation. There were considerable legal and administrative differences in the health and education services of the three countries of which any United Kingdom Training Council would have to take account.

Measures to ensure that a central council would be fully aware of national needs in the design of policy were contained in the second schedule to the Act. This required the Secretary of State to establish a Scottish Advisory Committee for each Council and set out its constitution. Section 8 of the same schedule gave the Minister of Health and Local Government in Northern Ireland similar powers. The first meeting of the Scottish Advisory Committee took place on 8 January 1963 under the chairmanship of Dr Nisbet, a member of Council. In Northern Ireland the committee was established one year later and met for the first time in September 1963 under the chairmanship of Professor Pemberton, a member of Council.

The importance of these committees was further emphasised by the fact that when the Council was first established, the Health Visitor Certificate was not required by regulation in either country. This followed in 1965[3] after considerable discussion between Government Departments, the committees and Council staff. As the name implies, neither advisory committee has executive powers, they exist to advise the Council on 'matters relating to exercise of its functions so far as they concern Scotland (or Northern Ireland)'. Administrative service is provided by the Scottish Home and Health Department and the Department of Health and Social Services in Northern Ireland.

Accounts of the business of each committee appeared in the periodic reports of the Council and therefore will not be repeated here. Reference will be found frequently to the particular needs of each country when main policy developments were discussed. One feature, however, which is not so easily demonstrated in a factual account is the more subtle influence of a 'forum for discussion', for the consideration of new ventures and the formation of contacts with related statutory bodies for nursing and midwifery in the countries concerned. Efforts were also made to design some joint activity with the advisory committees of the Social Work Council. In Scotland a joint seminar on the subject 'The Role of Health Visiting and Social Work in Relation to Primary Health Care' was held in 1970 while in Northern Ireland links were formed by ensuring some cross-membership of the two committees.

As the National Committees gained confidence in the use they might make of the main Council there was a change in attitude towards the concept of a United Kingdom body. Professional and administrative staff attended the advisory committees to answer questions and act as a further line of communication. When the Council was submitting its views to the Briggs Committee[4] on the statutory framework for nursing, midwifery and health visiting in 1970 and 1973, the pattern which had developed to ensure that all parts of the United Kingdom would receive due attention was warmly supported by both committees. In 1975 as a result of changes in authority in respect of Wales, the Council itself, on 19 March, set up a committee to give advice on the needs of the Principality.

THE COUNCIL AND THE GOVERNMENT DEPARTMENTS

In order to ensure a smooth beginning, decisions had to be made within the Government Departments upon the possible composition of the first Council committees. It would not have been practicable to await election by Council members as time was needed for them to become acquainted with each other. This distrust of appointed rather than elected councils and committees still exists and has been noted in some of the informal discussions taking place on the formation of new statutory bodies concerned with nursing, following the publication of the Briggs Report.[4] The physical separation of the Council from the Government Department premises and the appointment of its own secretariat was a major advance, but some distrust of Central Government particularly by the health visitor members, who in the first Council constituted more than one-third of its members, created something of a problem for the senior staff of the Council for the Training of Health Visitors. They were conscious of the need for strong support within the Government Departments if the Council's policy were to be effective but equally had to ensure that the various panels would not be unduly influenced by the presence of Government assessors. In time it was agreed that representatives of the Departments would be attending full Council meetings but not the small panels and committees. This implied a need to develop other kinds of communication with the Government Departments, a feature which has developed with the passage of time.

The first year generated great activity. In addition to frequent Council meetings, most members also served on one or more panels and the recurring contact which ensued produced a concentration of effort in preparing the new syllabus. The opportunity, in addition, of sharing panel discussions with representatives from the mainstream of education contributed greatly to the new approach to training. The experience was particularly stimulating to those health visitor members whose work had been restricted to a single vocational setting.

INTER-STAFF CONTACTS IN THE EARLY YEARS

A feature of sharing common resources among the Council officers was the impact of a closer relationship with colleagues from the field of social work. Although not necessarily in favour of the different approach to work and training of the social worker, their

greater independence in that they were developing a new qualification, as distinct from revising an existing certificate established
over many years, contributed, possibly unconsciously, to the thinking of the health visitor professional staff. At times the task of the
social work staff appeared infinitely simpler : no rigid first professional qualification for entering training; no restriction to one sex;
no inheritance of courses established over many years in employment situations; and above all, a topical public interest in social
work which resulted in a potentially large pool of recruitment.

This view of the Health Visitor Council's problem was not
shared by colleagues in Government Departments with the exception of some of the nursing officers. An observation was made to the
Chief Professional Advisor of the Health Visitor Council at the
end of her first year that the task must be a simple one as training
was already in being. The fact that what was established in 1925
was neither appropriate nor acceptable in 1962 did not appear to
be appreciated and the immensity of the task facing the Council
was probably not fully grasped by Government Departments,
Council members or even staff in the first instance.

Over the years, the professional staff increased from the original
three plus one Chief Professional Adviser, to six plus the Chief
Professional Adviser. This was matched by increases in the secretarial and office staff to carry the large administrative content of
the Council's statutory responsibility. These developments necessitated some expansion of offices to accommodate the new staff
and the Council leased further space in Clifton House. The
enlargement of staff and the increasing pace of work began to make
the original informal contact between the professional staff of
both Councils more erratic. For some time the health visitor staff
had organised an informal meeting once a month, to which professional colleagues from the Social Work Council and the senior
administrative staff were invited. Although it was possible to
maintain these gatherings for three years, the pressures of outside
commitments for all staff, administrative and professional, gradually made the arrangements more difficult and they were eventually
discontinued.

TRAINING FACILITIES IN 1962

Few situations arise in which it is possible to wipe the slate clean
and begin again. Reference has already been made to the inheritance from the training tradition of the nurse, i.e. learning on the
job, with those who are responsible for providing the service also
providing the training. Since the Council would require time to
formulate plans for the new training, it was agreed with The Royal
Society of Health and The Royal Sanitary Association of Scotland
that students would continue on the existing syllabus and enter the
appropriate examination as a temporary measure, i.e. for 1964 and
1965. Successful candidates would then acquire both the certificates of the examining body and of the Council. By this, 'blanket'
approval was given as an interim measure to all existing training
schools in order to provide for the continuation of training.[5]

In 1962, nineteen out of the twenty-seven existing training
schools were organised by employing authorities with widely differ-
ing facilities, in some cases related to university or technical
colleges but staffed by the Local Health Authority staff. There had
been no system of regular inspection, although in England and
Wales, nursing and medical officers from the Ministry of Health
visited at intervals. There was no comparable pattern in Scotland.
The visits from the Ministry of Health were related to the small
grant of £15 towards the fees of a course of six months and £25
towards a course of one year which was made for each individual
student by the Central Government Department.

The statutory responsibility for standards rested with the two
bodies, The Royal Society of Health and The Royal Sanitary
Association of Scotland, each of which laid down a syllabus and
conducted the central examination. They did not, however, normally visit the training centre and there was no common yardstick
against which an individual centre might either be assessed or seek
to measure its own performance. In many cases training was closely
associated with the need to staff an area and the costs of training
were absorbed into the general costs of the maternity and child
welfare service in which it was accepted the majority of the trainees
would be employed. Most candidates were sponsored[6] by Local

Health Authorities surrounding the city in which the training school was sited but there were a few independent candidates who, on conclusion of training, were free to apply for posts advertised in considerable numbers in the nursing journals.

The facilities available to students and tutors also varied. In some cases an arrangement had been reached with a university department or a local college of further education to provide class-room accommodation and some lectures. In few instances, however, were students part of the main student body, or their tutors part of the teaching staff of the establishment and consequently able to contribute to staff policy in the college. There was a slightly happier situation in two of the technical colleges where the staff were directly employed by the Education Authority. In general, such courses presented an appearance of two completely separate entities : e.g. in one university training school the professional staff of the Council saw students attending lectures in uniform and bringing their eleven o'clock coffee in flasks as they were not allowed to use the refectory. An inter-lecture break was taken in the classroom and they did not have access to the university library. Some training centres supplemented their resources with a small library and classroom in Local Authority premises. Where the training centres were organised entirely within the Local Health Authority, the official Head of the School might be the Medical Officer of Health but was more usually the medical officer responsible for the maternity and child welfare service or the superintendent health visitor. Conditions ranged widely : for example, one beautifully organised centre had individual rooms for tutorial staff in which to conduct small group work, light and well equipped classrooms, additional accommodation in which students might work on individual projects and comfortable common rooms in which they could prepare light meals. Here there were three tutorial staff to a total intake of approximately 20–25 students. At the other end of the scale there were training schools in which, for example, one tutor shared a large room with the entire student group at a considerable distance away from the Health Department. Some books were placed in a cupboard by way of a library. In another, partly disused premises were given to the centre with the major parts still used for general storage. Tutors and students were not in day-to-day touch with either Health or Education Authority staff.

There had been little attempt to establish the actual cost of providing the courses. Most authorities charged a fee, some as low as £10, although there was one interesting example, in which a group of authorities co-operated with a university assessing costs and distributing these among the participating authorities.

RECRUITMENT TO TRAINING IN 1962

The picture was not an optimistic one nor was it made any brighter by the small number of students entering training. Although it was still possible under the rules of The Royal Society of Health for candidates to complete a four year course leading to the examination for the certificate without previous registration as a nurse,[7] this particular form of training had fallen into disuse due to lack of candidates. Most Local Health Authorities asked that applicants for a post in their service should be nurses on the general register and some also asked that they should be State Certified Midwives. This had implications for the recruitment of health visitor students in the absence of a coherent policy on recruitment to the whole nursing service whether hospital or community.

Individual hospitals obtained student nurses to meet their own requirements and literature designed to attract to the nursing profession by Government Departments or independent publishers emphasised the clinical aspects of the training period and placed little emphasis on career prospects in general. This not only presented a biased picture to the potential nurse, it did not indicate to her parents or teachers the opportunities open to her after registration. The attention of the National Consultative Committee for Recruitment of Nurses and Midwives was drawn to this after the Council had been invited to join that Committee in January 1964. This limitation to the hospital field did affect somewhat the variety of candidates recruited to nursing. In addition, the Council was faced with the problem of ensuring that information on health visitor courses reached the nurse once she had embarked upon training. The formation of a special group to examine this was agreed at the Council meeting in December 1963.[8]

REFERENCES

1 *An Inquiry into Health Visiting* (Jameson Report), HMSO 1956.
2 *CTHV Proceedings of Council,* HV/M/1 (25.10.62).
3 The National Health Service (Qualification of Health Visitors) (Scotland) Regulations 1965 SI 1965 No. 1490 (S.80). Qualification of Health Visitors 1965 Statutory Rules and Orders of Northern Ireland 1965 No. 1.
4 *Report of the Committee on Nursing.* Chairman: Professor Asa Briggs. Cmnd. 5115. HMSO 1972.
5 *CTHV Proceedings of Council,* HV/M/9 (13.1.64).
6 A 'sponsored' candidate usually received a proportion, e.g. two-thirds or three-quarters of a health visitor's first year salary while training. Most authorities required the student to give an undertaking to work in the authority concerned for one to two years on completing training. There was no uniform system. A fuller description may be found in CTHV *Evidence to the Committee on Nursing,* December 1970.
7 Royal Society of Health, *Regulations and Syllabus for the Examinations for Health Visitors in England and Wales,* 1950.
8 *CTHV Proceedings of Council* HV/M/8 (2.12.63).

Chapter 3

ESTABLISHING THE POLICY

I 'spect I growd
Topsy in *Uncle Tom's Cabin*—HARRIET BEECHER STOWE

FINANCIAL CONSTRAINTS AND NEW TRAINING OBJECTIVES

The Council was faced with the problem of ensuring a continued supply of recruits to an already established statutory service while at the same time attempting to supply a more realistic and appropriate training. The task was not made easier by the financial arrangements under which the Council operated. Although there had been much debate during the passage of the Bill through the House on the question of financial support, no central funds were placed at Council's disposal for either the upgrading of training centres or for the training of an adequate number of tutors.[1] In 1963 there were thirty-eight health visitor tutors in post who possessed a certificate of teacher training. In the case of the Social Work Council the position was somewhat easier in that the National Institute for Social Work Training, a voluntary body with a general interest in the development of training, had access to Trust Funds and was able to provide for the training of their first tutors.

The tradition in nursing as a whole that training must accompany the provision of service rather than precede it and therefore should be incorporated in the service budget held good for health visitors. Although the majority of students had, nominally at least, no service commitments during their training period a number of authorities expected the training to be so arranged that the students' timetable appeared to match that of employed staff with only the public holidays to break the length of the course. The quality of service which could be given by a student not actually based in an area as a permanent member of staff and attending only at intervals due to the exigencies of the classroom instruction was seldom appreciated. Rather, efforts were made to compress the theoretical teaching into defined compartments so that the student was presented with two distinct sections to her course, i.e. learning in the centre and practice in the employing authorities.

The Council saw obvious problems in laying down a formal policy in relation to training. It would have been possible, theoretically at least, to have declared a moratorium on any change for a period of some years while an ideal system was designed. Indeed at an early stage one of the professional associations felt that there would be value in deferring any legislation on health visitor training. The Council decided, however, not to delay for a number of reasons. It accepted with great seriousness its responsibilities for maintaining a constant flow of effectively trained health visitors into the service. There were advantages in allowing for modification in the light of experience and dangers in creating an inflexible pattern incapable of adaptation and advance. The Council members were also very conscious of the part played by most authorities in providing training in the past. This had often been done under extremely difficult circumstances and the medical and nursing staff concerned had made some notable contributions. A protracted discussion leading to a long delay in planning new training would have been a poor reward to those who had worked hard to improve training within previous constraints.

The Council, therefore, attempted to achieve a flexible system in its formulation of policy. While at times it may have appeared to resemble that of Topsy, it was in fact not unplanned, indeed, it was designed to achieve progress within the limitations of the position existing in 1962. The two panels considering syllabus and examination and fieldwork respectively made their recommendations to Council which accepted these at their ninth meeting on 13 January 1964[2].

The decisions concerning the training appeared revolutionary but were the rational outcome of considering both ends and means. The membership of the two panels who made the recommendations contained wide representation from universities, further education, medicine, nursing administration and health visitor tutors as well as members of the employing authorities. The Council had thought that the first approach to a new training might be best achieved by an examination of the current employment of the health visitor but although it had been hoped to achieve this by distributing a questionnaire to Local Health Authorities it proved very difficult to reach agreement on a suitable design. Eventually, more simply, a letter was sent to Council members seeking information on the nature of the work in their own setting.[3] This in effect produced a description of health visitor activity in a considerable number of Local Health Authorities in the United Kingdom. Unfortunately, however, not only the actual work varied from area to area, so also did its description. Previous revisions of the syllabus had come up against this stumbling block of diverse forms of practice and the Panel on Syllabus and Examination Procedure therefore decided to attempt a more fundamental approach by identifying areas of study which would provide a knowledge base from which could stem the current topics.

THE RELATIONSHIP BETWEEN PRE-REGISTRATION COURSES AND SUBSEQUENT HEALTH VISITOR TRAINING

The decision was also made that it would grow out of general nurse training and a period of experience in obstetric nursing or midwifery. Although training in some form of nursing along with midwifery or maternity nursing experience had been one of the preconditions for entry to health visitor training for many years, the nature of the relationship of the three trainings was not clear. When the Council took office it was still possible for a candidate to offer registration as a Sick Children's Nurse in England and Wales as a suitable preparation for admission to health visitor training.[4] The first part of the midwifery course had been considered acceptable for many years and the incorporation of an obstetric nurse placement within some of the integrated courses for state registration and health visiting and the later extension of this to an option within general training had also been approved. There was a need now to regulate the position. Just as the syllabus should show a logical progression so in its turn there should be a logical progression from previous training. Too often in the past there had been insufficient emphasis on the background obtained from general nursing in the teaching of health visiting. In the view of the Council an understanding of the processes of disease was an important element in the health visitor's preparation.

In deciding that this would be best obtained through preparation for the general register the Panel was influenced by changes in nurse training. In England there had been revision of that syllabus in 1952 and during 1960–61 the Education Committee of the General Nursing Council for England and Wales prepared a draft syllabus with a 'new look'. It would have three main sections :

1. The principles and practice of nursing including first aid.
2. The study of the human individual.
3. Concepts of the nature and cause of disease and the principles of prevention and treatment.[5]

In Scotland plans to phase out the decision to abolish special registers and consequently to provide a comprehensive training was made in 1967 (although these were not implemented) but discussion on this possibility had been taking place for some years and since 1963 a three week programme of teaching on Local Health Authority work had been included in the general training of the nurse.

The potential breadth of the training in both countries upon which the health visitor course could build was now ready to be exploited. This was particularly opportune as the health visitor's concern for all age groups in the community was growing. The decision was therefore made that candidates should no longer be admitted to training from the special registers and the specially designed course of four years which only included a short period of nursing experience would no longer be recognised.[6]

This decision to base the health visitor training on general and obstetric nursing was highly significant for later developments. It committed the Council to the acceptance of health visiting as part of nursing and it is possible that the implications for the future of this decision were not entirely understood at the time. Discussion described in Chapter 5 demonstrates the ambivalent position in which many Council members found themselves. The step taken in 1964 led inevitably to the incorporation of the Council in the revision of the Nursing and Midwifery Councils proposed by the Briggs Committee in 1970.

THE FIELDWORK ELEMENT IN A REVISED TRAINING PROGRAMME

There were considerable difficulties in a realistic design of syllabus which could be covered in a limited period. It must be remembered that in 1962 training could be completed within six months and although with few exceptions, it was accepted that there would be extension to an academic year, there was real anxiety that a longer course would seem unattractive to candidates who had already spent not less than four years in professional training. Early discussion in the Education Committee centred round the possibility of adding a substantial period of practical work after college and before certification.[7] Eventually it was decided that there should be a short continuous period of supervised practice, making the course one calendar year and that in order to fit with normal college arrangements this would generally be from July to September.

This immediately raised other questions : for example, what sort of areas should provide the experience? Was it appropriate to use those in which triple duties were carried out by one worker? What sort of staff should carry out supervision? In 1965, the Council refused to accept as suitable for supervision, an area in which there was no superintendent nursing officer at all, and where the health visiting staff came under the direct control of one of the staff of the Medical Officer of Health.[8]

A study carried out by the Council's staff to assist the work of the Recruitment Committee[9] found that in a number of authorities there was no superintendent nursing officer and it was appreciated that Council might well lay down requirements about supervision which it would be impossible to carry out. Once more the Council was faced with the problem of either designing a training which would, hopefully, provide candidates for the future and an improved working situation or limiting the horizon to what was available at the moment. It was decided to follow the former plan, but the developments were not without difficulties.

UTILISING NEW RESOURCES

The last revisions of the syllabus had been made in 1950 by The Royal Society of Health and in 1956 by The Royal Sanitary Association of Scotland. The Council's Panel had to take account of the advances in medicine, in social and behavioural sciences, the resources which might be available for teaching outside the health departments and the impact of new colleagues in the Health and Welfare Services, i.e. the social workers for whom their sister Council was established. The objective now was to design a syllabus of four to five sections which would provide a framework of study which would not necessarily change over the years but would permit modifications in the light of changes in the service, along with an introduction of new techniques and work. An explanation of the rationale and the design was given in the Council's First Report and developed further in Guide to Syllabus of Training.

Before putting its new concept into practice the Council invited a few training schools to interpret the prototype syllabus by designing a curriculum which would be practicable within their own facilities. As in the nurse training school, where the greater part of teaching is carried out by the tutorial and medical staff of hospitals concerned, health visitor training centres had tended to rely heavily on the staff of the Local Health Authority within whose area the centre was situated. Some lecturers might contribute to teaching but be established within an adjacent educational institution which took no part in the final examination although they might be involved in setting and marking internal test papers. The health visitor tutors who co-operated in preparing draft curricula were asked to bear in mind the possibility of drawing upon the knowledge and expertise of non-medical teachers of the behavioural and social sciences for lecture series. This widened the range of teachers

with whom health visitor students would have contact and introduced the possibility of some shared work with other students.

FACTORS IN THE DESIGN
OF THE NEW SYLLABUS

The idea of providing a common base for a variety of vocations
was receiving considerable attention in the sixties. A report of the
Institute for Social Research[10] advocated a basic preparation which
would, in addition to providing pre-clinical training for the medical
student, allow for shared training with other workers such as nurses
and social workers. Experience in the Diploma of Community
Nursing (later the degree of Bachelor of Nursing) of the University
of Manchester demonstrated the practicability of providing a
theoretical base in, for example, psychology, social anthropology
and social administration in common with other students. These
subjects served to add weight to the vocational element in the total
course.[11]

In designing the sections in the new syllabus, the Council
followed a logical progression from study of the human life-cycle
to the social and cultural factors influencing growth and development; consideration of the social policy of our society; the actual
service, organisation and current medical problems with which the
Health Service was concerned and finally study of the health
visitor's particular contribution and the techniques she might
employ. The interesting possibility which emerged from this new
approach to designing a syllabus was that of more consistent sharing of teaching. The first three sections covered areas of concern
to a number of workers in the caring professions. This development
contributed to the later work of the Joint Advisory Committee of
the two Councils in which members explored the common ground
as well as the differences between health visitors and social workers.

A NEW APPROACH TO THE EXAMINATION

Having agreed the subjects of study, the Panel on Syllabus and
Examination Procedure had to give consideration to the ways in
which these might be examined. As the certificate was required by

Statute, the Council, as the responsible body, had to ensure an acceptable standard. The examination in 1962 was organised centrally, although The Royal Society of Health in England had asked training schools to arrange facilities for their own students and a similar arrangement pertained to Scotland. There are arguments both for and against a centrally organised system. It does ensure that where all students have passed through the same procedure the standard achieved will be national rather than local. It has to be remembered, however, that just as the number of musicians with perfect pitch is small, even smaller must be the number of examiners who can carry within them the perfect standard which will not be affected by the nature of the group to which it is to be applied. If an attempt is made to lay down a standard which be will appropriate over, for example, the United Kingdom, this may well be a minimum and may not encourage the gradual improvement in quality of learning and teaching which a training body would seek to achieve.

The Panel members were convinced that the examination should be a logical outcome of the teaching programme, that it should become more specific by consisting of papers set on the various sections of the syllabus and therefore that lecturers not previously participating would now become involved in the examination procedure. In making this decision the Council was well aware of the criticism which might be levelled at the new pattern and as the years progressed was prepared to consider to what extent some common standard was being achieved and eventually, as is described in Chapter 7, set up a research investigation to see in what way variation is taking place in the standards reached in the various training schools.

INTRODUCTION OF THE FIELDWORK TEACHER

Previous revision of syllabus had always been related to a theoretical aspect of training but the need to improve and to some extent standardise the content and quality of the accompanying fieldwork practice had been recognised by many tutors. A panel to consider the fieldwork of the health visitor student was established at the first meeting of the Council and reported at the same time as the Panel on the Syllabus and Examination Procedure. Its task was peculiarly difficult. While it might be possible to lay down criteria for practice, the Council had no powers under the Act to enforce standards on staff not within their own employment. Under the previous system a few training schools had made a small payment either to the health visitors accepting their students by agreement with the employing authority or directly to the Local Health Authority concerned. This allowed the schools concerned to exercise some choice in the selection of those health visitors contributing to training. The practice had, however, been declining, particularly after the introduction of the National Health Service in 1948 when the responsibility for maternity and child welfare service passed from the small authorities to the County Boroughs and County Councils.

As with all the changes proposed by the Council the fieldwork proposals were influenced by procedures and changes taking place in other fields. The need to designate and prepare a nurse specifically for practical teaching in the ward situation had been recognised. Development began in Scotland and by 1962 the Scottish General Nursing Council was empowered to grant recognition to clinical teachers.[12] The Royal College of Nursing in London introduced courses for clinical teachers in 1963 and the General Nursing Council for England and Wales was allowed some money to finance their training, although the next step, i.e. that of registration, was not approved by the Ministry of Health.[13] In other countries, for example in certain schools in the United States of America, the clinical teacher is a member of staff of the training institution and obtains facilities for work with individual families or patients by agreement with the Local Health Department. Such a development in this country would have allowed the training schools to exercise very much greater control over the nature of the actual practical instruction. They could have ensured that the teachers joining their staff were appropriately prepared and that there would be careful selection of the material to be taught. On the other hand the situation would have been highly artificial. The Panel, although anxious to deepen the health visitor's capacity and quality of perception in dealing with individual problems, was also concerned that she would learn how to determine priorities within the very wide range of the work presented to her as a general health visitor.

The members were convinced that there must be some system of selecting practical teachers who had not merely a capacity to work well as health visitors, but also the ability to analyse work so as to assist the student to learn from it. Other factors to be borne in mind were the presence of staff in some areas with responsibility for the triple duties of midwifery, district nursing and health visiting and, overall, the difficulties of ensuring appropriate supervision.

CRITERIA FOR THE ACCEPTANCE OF FIELDWORK AREAS

After the new training system had been accepted by the Council, a letter setting out the requirements was sent to Local Health Authorities on 20 December 1966.

The student remains the responsibility of the Health Visitor Training Centre until the end of the calendar year. The student may undertake her continuous period of experience in her sponsoring authority provided:

1. She is able to undertake whole time health visiting (triple duties would not be considered appropriate experience in this instance).
2. That there is a superintendent nursing officer in the Local Health Authority and that there are adequate intermediate supervisory staff to assist the student with advice on the management of her area.
3. The area concerned should have a very small case load, approximately 100 families.
4. The student can return to training school during the period. The arrangements will vary with the individual school but a suggested plan is that the student returns approximately once a month. It will be obvious, therefore, that she must be within reasonable travelling distance for this purpose.

The training school will arrange for a period of vacation at the beginning or end of the continuous practice.

Any attempt to establish the actual content of fieldwork was even more difficult. Ostensibly health visitors were employed to meet the requirements of the National Health Service Act.[14]

In practice health visitors were deployed to meet local need but this could be affected by the vision or personal interest of the Medical Officer of Health or the tradition of the employing authorities. It was clear that improvement could only be achieved by a gradual process. The Panel, however, was able to begin to differentiate between real practice with its development of skills and the provision of simple observation of a variety of services. This involved it in an attempt to identify the skills, a process which only came to fruition later in the work done on the function of the health visitor to be explored in Chapter 5.

The Council was under some pressure, which still continues, to include preparation both in the classroom and the field in specific screening procedures, the most usual being the assessment of hearing in the young child. A number of Local Authorities operated such assessment and screening schemes. In the opinion of the Panel it should be possible to design curricula on the new syllabus which would incorporate current techniques without listing these specifically. A detailed and specific list could lead to the teaching of procedures no longer in common use, although possibly still used in a few areas, always a problem when a syllabus is established.

THE FIELDWORK CONTENT OF THE EXAMINATION

The Panel was hoping to achieve close integration of theory and practice and therefore to include assessment of practical ability in the examination system. In the past examiners had relied on hypothetical questions in the oral examination as well as similar examples in the written papers, to test the candidate's ability to apply her understanding of theory to a practical situation. A way had to be found by which the potential health visitor could demonstrate the development of her understanding over a period of contact with actual families and this led to the novelty of the 'family studies' (now known as 'health visiting studies'). These were to consist of contact during the academic year with four families or individuals who might illustrate some aspect of the health visitor's work, for example, advice and help to the mother of a new baby, surveying the development of toddlers or school children, assessing the health and environment of an elderly person either living alone or in a family, or an individual member of a family with a disability and the needs inherent in the situation. The student would visit her 'families' at intervals and provide a record of contact and work. This would not merely be a simple narrative account, it would illustrate the student's capacity to form an elementary assessment on her first contact with the family, the setting of priorities in her subsequent visiting and her evaluation at the end of progress achieved. Such a study could obviously include any of the current screening procedures used in relation to the families concerned and was likely to provide a much more practical and meaningful illustration than demonstration of these in a classroom situation. To deepen the skill further the Panel considered that there should be study of a particular aspect of work to be presented at the final examination either as a project or in a day book. The latter was little used but the projects developed. Students, as well as examiners, were able to use this method as a means of assessment. A random choice of four titles from one school indicates the variety of interests pursued.

  (i) Toy libraries;

 (ii) A study of self-help treatment used by mothers for infant teething disturbance;

(iii) Educational opportunities for a haemophiliac boy;

(iv) 'And some gave them brown'—domiciliary meals and luncheon clubs for the elderly.

During this discussion it was becoming clear that the arbitrary division into two panels, one considering syllabus and the other practical work, was artificial and the two panels therefore came together and reported at the same time to the Council (see p. 22).

THE MOVE TO EDUCATIONAL INSTITUTIONS

A number of consequences of the new training will be noted. If the curriculum derived from the new syllabus was to draw upon resources other than those which could be provided by the Health Authority it followed that there must be a greater reliance on educational establishments. If students were to be encouraged to consider their service in relation to the needs of the community as a whole they needed to have an opportunity for freer discussion with students from other disciplines, preparation for work in the community and have access to a wide range of books and journals. The course would have to be designed to help them develop a critical faculty and an ability to set goals and objectives in the service they provide. It was obvious, therefore, that the growth of facilities in colleges and university departments was not only to be fostered but actively promoted.

It was fortuitous but nevertheless particularly fortunate that the Council's policy coincided with the growth of resources in further education generally and the Council was able to take advantage of this expansion. Development of policy, therefore, was an admixture of the fashioning of a new philosophy and the exploitation of current resources. The form the policy took allowed for later development, some of which has materialised, for example the acceptance of alternative qualifications. The design of special courses for the certificate for candidates from other countries was an outcome of this. Other developments which might have been expected to be a natural consequence of a syllabus which shared certain common elements with that of other vocations, the teaching for which could be provided in departments which housed a range of courses, have not unfortunately taken place to any great extent.

AN EDUCATIONAL STANDARD FOR ENTRANTS

More criticism was engendered by the recommendation that candidates should have a defined educational standard. At the time the Council was instituted some training schools included an estimate of educational ability when interviewing candidates. Although student selection had been discussed in the Standing Conference of Health Visitor Training Centres from time to time, the methods used in training schools varied and just as there was no clear definition of skills to be developed during the health visitors' course, so no clear definition of prerequisite ability existed. Much importance in the past had been placed on the selection interview.

Florence Nightingale once made the acid comment 'We are often told that a nurse needs only to be "devoted and obedient". This definition . . . might even do for a horse.'[15] An early job description in one city for health visitor candidates in the twenties required that they should be 'between 25 and 35 years of age, unmarried, healthy and good walkers', and one might be tempted to assume that in the sixties the possession of physical stamina was still considered of greater importance than intellectual ability. The health visitor whose function had been defined as that of 'health education and social advice' obviously must be skilled in communication and in this one of her most important tools would be her command of language.

The Panel on Syllabus and Examination Procedure accepted in discussion that, while it would be possible in the course of an academic year to develop a potential already present, it would not be realistic to make good early shortcomings in education. It would also not be possible to impose a capacity for easy communication on students who had not demonstrated some such ability in previous occupations. To continue to accept candidates without this basic skill was damaging to the service and, even more important, to the self-respect of the individual thus exposed to the likelihood of failure both academically and in the formation of her relationships. Much has been written and debated on the value of the General Certificate of Education by experts in education, by employers and by the public at large. It could be argued that a certificate obtained at the age of sixteen does not necessarily give a satisfactory forecast of ability some ten or fifteen years later by which time a whole range of social skills and abilities are required. Nevertheless it can be regarded as a statement of subjects studied to a general standard when listed as a prerequisite and can also be useful as an indication to others of the type of course to be followed. The Council, therefore, accepted that candidates in future should possess the General Certificate of Education with five passes at Ordinary level and specified some of the subjects to be covered.[16] Where candidates did not possess such a certificate the college was required to provide some form of educational assessment and the process being used would be submitted as part of the approval system when the proposal for training was being submitted to the Council.

OBSTETRIC NURSING AS A PREREQUISITE EXPERIENCE

Health visiting originated as a service for mothers and babies and the contribution to the antenatal service through health education as well as the actual management of clinic services required a knowledge of midwifery. For this, health visitor training had in the past relied upon the certificates gained prior to the health visitor course. Now the nature of the obstetric nurse experience occupied much debate. The Standing Conference of Health Visitor Training Centres had promoted discussion on this part of health visitor preparation. In general, comment on the nature of the first part of the midwifery training was highly critical. But it was all too easy to criticise the existing training and to forget it had not been designed specifically for the potential health visitor. It was therefore only an administrative convenience to rely upon a form of preparation for which the health visitor training body had no responsibility. It would have been possible to design an appropriate course within that of the Health Visitor Certificate, but this would inevitably have led to a longer course which was unlikely to be acceptable. Although the majority of health visitors courses covered the academic year, at the time of the Council's inception there were still two which could be completed in six and seven months respectively. While it was accepted that these could not continue and that nine months would be required, the further steps which the Council took in 1964[17] to extend the course to a calendar year, in order to provide a satisfactory amount of practical teaching, led to great opposition.

With the recognition, therefore, that there is a limit to the amount of change which can be tolerated in any one period, the

Council accepted the recommendation of the two Panels and in 1965 the new system of training was introduced. The syllabus indicated broad areas of study and absorbed approximately two-thirds of the academic year. Fieldwork was to be supervised by specialist staff to be known as fieldwork instructors and should concentrate on actual practical experience. The examination would be the responsibility of the individual training schools which would be based in an appropriate educational institution. It should include three written papers, four studies of families with whom the student had been associated during the year and a project on a chosen topic.

All candidates for training should have a standard educational background and those who might have completed their education some years earlier and who had not obtained recognised certificates should pass a test set and administered by the training school and approved by the Council. All candidates should be on the general register of the General Nursing Councils, should be either State Certified Midwives, have taken Part I Midwifery Training or should have obtained obstetric nursing experience in courses recognised by the Central Midwives' Board of either country.

FACILITIES FOR GRADUATE CANDIDATES

As time progressed and the Council's activities in relation to recruitment bore fruit (Chapter 6) there followed the establishment of new courses in a number of areas and the overall entry to training increased (Appendix III). Although this presented an encouraging picture, the Council was concerned that a number of good candidates were not accommodated in the system, e.g. graduates of the nursing degree courses both from the United Kingdom and abroad, the older candidates with some family responsibilities and the triple duty nurses working without health visitor qualifications, mainly in Scotland.

Many of the nurse graduates had already covered some major parts of the syllabus. Accordingly, training schools were invited to submit details of such applicants to see if remission of part of the syllabus could be allowed. The colleges were also encouraged to design extended courses, i.e. covering two years instead of one to meet the needs of the older candidate who might wish to work at a more leisurely pace either because she had not undertaken study for a number of years, or because she had to maintain some family commitments.

SPECIAL COURSE FOR TRIPLE DUTY NURSES IN SCOTLAND

Finally, in order to meet the particular needs of Scotland, a special course for working nurses was designed for a limited number of intakes. This course made use of daily work as fieldwork and covered some of the theory by means of special assignments to be completed at home. It therefore made considerable concessions as the candidates were usually engaged in duties which covered district midwifery and district nursing in addition. Normally this would not have been acceptable as fieldwork since the total health visiting content may be small. The proposal was greeted with enthusiasm by some nursing officers concerned at the number of their staff working without certificates. The actual proportion of staff seconded to this experimental training has however been very disappointing.[18] Nevertheless the exercise has demonstrated the Council's willingness to produce a scheme to meet special needs and has dispelled views of it as a rigid and inflexible body. A second and somewhat unexpected effect has been the increased number of entrants to orthodox training from the areas traditionally associated with problems of staffing.

REFERENCES

1 HC Debate (1961–62) 665, c.1697.
  HC Debate (1961–62) 665, c.16.
  HC Debate (1961–62) 665, c.6w.
2 The two panels referred to were: the Panel on Syllabus and Examination Procedure (Chairman: Professor T. E. Chester) and the Panel on Practical Work Supervision (Chairman: Miss D. J. Lamont).
3 *CTHV Proceedings of Council*, HV/M/3 (4.3.63).
4 The Royal Society of Health, *Regulations and Syllabus for the Examinations for Health Visitors in England and Wales, 1950.*
5 The syllabus was introduced in 1962 as an experimental syllabus and it became compulsory five years later. Discussions with the Central

Midwives Board had already begun in 1959 to widen obstetric experience in general training; the first courses commenced in 1961. By 1971 training for the general part of the Register had been widened to include one of the following: psychiatric or geriatric or obstetric nursing or community care. From January 1975 two of the following were required: either psychiatric or geriatric nursing and either obstetric or community care.

6 HV/M/9 (13.1.64).

7 *CTHV Proceedings of Education Committee* HV/EC/M/3 (2.10.64).

8 *CTHV Proceedings of Education Committee* HV/EC/M/6 (21.1.65).

9 *CTHV Proceedings of Recruitment Committee* HV/RC/67/2 (19.1.67). Appendix (d).

10 Institute for Social Research 1967. *A Comprehensive Medical School.*

11 Brockington, F. *A University Course in Nursing,* The University of Manchester 1969.

12 Nurses (Scotland) (Amendment No. 2) Rules 1961. Approval Instrument 1962.

13 Bendall, E. R. D. and Raybould, E. *History of the General Nursing Council 1919–1969,* H. K. Lewis 1969.

14 National Health Service Act 1946, 9 and 10 Geo. 6. Ch. 81.
Part III, Section 24.
(1) It shall be the duty of every local health authority to make provision in its area for the visiting of persons in their homes by visitors, to be called 'health visitors' for the purpose of giving advice as to the care of young children, persons suffering from illness and expectant or nursing mothers, and to the measures necessary to prevent the spread of infection.
(2) The duty of a local authority under this section may be discharged by making arrangements with voluntary organisations for the employment by those organisations of health visitors or by themselves employing health visitors.

15 Nightingale, F. *Notes on Nursing,* first published 1859 (Hamson and Sons). Reissued 1952 (Duckworth).

16 CTHV Training Rules. Rule 4 (ii) (c) 1965.

17 CTHV Training Rules.

18 A special course for uncertificated health visitors was approved for five intakes and was started in Dundee in 1972. It is now discontinued.

Chapter 4

ESTABLISHING THE NEW STANDARD

> If you want style, madam, you must pay for it.
> (Shop assistant to impecunious customer)

The mere introduction of a new syllabus will not of itself raise standards of training or practice. Any advance must be paid for by acceptance of change as well as by actual money. The important feature of the new Council was its power to develop standards in the implementation of any such syllabus. There were various means by which it might achieve this. First the Council had authority, it laid down Rules under which training might be carried out and these were approved by the Health Ministers.[1] The Council granted approval to training schools directly, it did not make a recommendation to the Health Ministers as did the previous bodies. Under the Act it could provide further training for health visitors where this was lacking or insufficient. The Council could seek to attract suitable persons to training and lastly it could undertake research or promote research activities into the training of health visitors.

THE PROFESSIONAL STAFF, INSPECTOR OR ADVISER?

The other great resource at the disposal of the Council which had not been available to the Royal Society of Health and The Royal Sanitary Association of Scotland was an establishment of professional staff. The title given to the main grade, i.e. 'Adviser' should be noted. Although professional organisations may campaign for some regulation of standards many of their members may fear the introduction of 'Inspection'. Indeed this fear extends to the lay public. It was only after prolonged debate that the General Nursing Council for England and Wales, established in 1919, was able to introduce a limited system of inspection carried out by Council members and it was not until 1939 that this was extended to include the Local Authority hospitals. It was 1944 before the General Nursing Council was given permission to appoint salaried staff for this purpose.[2] The term 'Inspector', however, unfairly implies criticism and interference. It is not known why the word 'Adviser' was used for the new Council, but it was interpreted by the first professional staff as indicating a liberal approach to their contact with schools; although appointed as advisers to the Council they were freely consulted by course organisers and from the outset their effort was directed towards working together with their tutor colleagues to raise standards. It may be noted that although in 1962 a number of training schools were operating with most inadequate resources in regrettable surroundings, no school has ever had approval withdrawn by the decision of the Council on these grounds.

The provision of an Advisory Service must in its turn have a firm framework. In addition to its powers under the Act to lay down formal Rules the Council drew up a guide to these Rules.[1]

The training schools therefore had some very general directions. It is not possible to provide for all eventualities, however carefully worded, some interpretation of these Rules to the local situation is always required. In the first instance this was in part covered by the professional staff visits. It was at a later date that a Handbook for the use of schools was designed.[3] The establishment of the three professional advisers did not occur until October 1964 but in the period of July 1963 to July 1964 the Chief Professional Adviser succeeded in visiting all the existing training schools, some more than once, where there were particular problems, and one or two cities where there was interest in the development of new training schools.

These visits were planned to introduce the new training body, to discuss the nature of its contact with the schools and to build up knowledge on existing conditions, a regular system for the future had to be allowed to develop more slowly. In addition to the natural distrust individuals might have of officialdom (however well known the first holder of the post of Chief Professional Adviser might have been to her professional colleagues), there were several reasons for allowing development to proceed somewhat cautiously. The Council had to establish its image as a responsible, forward-looking body in the eyes of the Local Authorities both Health and Education. The relationship with the former was particularly delicate. The Council laid great emphasis on the practical nature of the new training and was therefore dependent upon the goodwill of the Local Health Authorities for teaching facilities. A difficulty was created by the decision that teaching must be undertaken by designated teachers.[4] In Local Government, there is always concern lest authority be eroded by Central Government Departments. Although the Council was not a section of any such department, its powers stemmed from an Act, it operated centrally and its responsibilities extended over the United Kingdom. Its decisions were therefore likely to be questioned almost as a matter of principle.

IMPLICATIONS OF LACK OF CENTRAL FUNDS FOR TRAINING

Undoubtedly the Council's task would have been greatly eased if it had been given the financial resources to establish courses for fieldwork instructors and to distribute, possibly through the training schools, grants to such instructors. This dependence by the Council on resources controlled by other bodies was a constant problem throughout the twelve years under review, and was one of the major obstacles to more rapid progress in the appropriate training of health visitor tutors. It compared unfavourably, in this sense, both with the General Nursing Council which was able to provide finance for both sister tutors and clinical instructors and with facilities for the child care courses operated through the Home Office in which the entire cost of the training was borne by the Central Government Department. The need for financial support both to students and to courses in view of the need to meet a considerable shortfall in health visitors and social workers was raised during the debate on the Training Bill, but in both written and oral answer the principle of central support was not accepted.[5] Looking back it is difficult to see why so few resources were made available to the Council in view of the task it faced.

As the quality of training depends in its turn on the quality of the teaching within the courses, there must be adequate facilities for the preparation of tutors and of fieldwork teachers. In the *Guide to the Training Rules* (1965) it is stated that, in granting approval to a training course the Council would expect there to be not less than one health visitor tutor for every fifteen students over and above other teaching staff. The proportion of fieldwork teachers should be one to two or three students. Although a few training centres had such a staff/student ratio, the great majority had a much lower ratio and few had organised fieldwork teachers.

TUTOR TRAINING

The first course for health visitor tutors was established by the Royal College of Nursing in conjunction with the City of Birmingham Health Department in 1948. The Standing Conference of Health Visitor Training Centres had been concerned for some time at the lack of systematic preparation for teachers of health visitors. This concern increased during the expansion of training centres after 1948 which focused attention on the need to safeguard the quality of the teaching. The next step after the provision of a course leading to a certificate was the institution of a Roll of holders of appropriate qualifications and this was set up by the Royal College of Nursing in 1953. Admission was not limited to holders of the College's certificate, applications were accepted from holders of other specified teaching qualifications provided there had also been experience for three years as a whole time health visitor. As happens frequently this pioneer work by a professional organisation led at a later date to assumption of responsibility by a statutory body. The expansion of health visitor training into the mainstream of higher and further education and the availability of technical teacher courses in four institutions in England increased the variety of course and qualification open to the health visitor interested in developing her career in student training. On the 28 June 1967, therefore, the Council took over responsibility for the Roll, which at that time contained 108 names.

Efforts to increase the numbers of tutors encountered obstacles. For the first tutor course in 1948 the Ministry of Health and the Scottish Home and Health Department had offered a total of twelve scholarships. These, however, were not repeated; it was expected that the Local Health Authorities, at that time mainly responsible for the training centres, would second staff for tutor training when required thereafter. In most cases, however, this resulted in appointment from within the staff of the authority concerned. Not only did this foster a narrow and parochial approach to training but also it offered no opportunity to the able health visitor working in an authority which did not possess a training school. For some years competitive scholarships were offered by charitable organisations[6] and a number of tutors were able to obtain financial support in this way.

The obvious solution would have been a small number of grants to be offered on a competitive basis each year from a central source. Despite repeated discussions it was not possible to reach a satisfactory solution. An attempt was made in 1966 to improve matters by the issue of circulars to Local Health Authorities by the Government Department. In these, authorities were reminded of the 'pooling'[7] of finance for health visitor and tutor training and were strongly encouraged to make full use of such resources. By this system those authorities who had spent money on health visitor training would have this taken into account when their Rate Support Grant was computed. Theoretically this should have spread the burden of expense more evenly among all authorities : in practice the results were not completely satisfactory in that there was no direct recompense to the Public Health Department as such. A small increase in tutor students followed, but unfortunately was not maintained.

The impact of the new requirements was, of course, felt more directly by medical officers of health and superintendent health visitors and the introduction of the fieldwork instructor aroused great controversy, in part related to the introduction of a new grade, and in part to the concept of supervising up to three students. The Medical Officer of Health was disturbed by the financial implications, the Superintendent Health Visitor by the possible division of loyalties while the field health visitor tended to construe this novelty both as a slur on her capacity to teach her own speciality and on the value of the one-to-one relationship with the student. The recommendation that a fieldwork instructor might be responsible for more than one student was intended to develop some interplay of interest among two or three students which would illuminate all their work, while the reduction in the actual number of health visitors undertaking practical instruction would allow a greater degree of concentration of the skills of practical teaching on a selected minority.

PREPARING THE FIELDWORK TEACHERS

Since no direct funds were available some means had to be found whereby training could be instituted for fieldwork instructors within existing provisions. For some years health visitors had been able to attend refresher courses at intervals of five years as part of conditions of service. These were usually two weeks in length and fees, subsistence and any necessary travelling expenses could be paid by the employing authority. Although this provision applied to England and Wales only, a number of the more enlightened Health Authorities in Scotland had sent staff to short courses provided by the Royal College of Nursing from time to time. The pattern of releasing staff for study leave was accepted. The Council therefore invited those organisations providing the majority of refresher course places, along with any training schools willing to co-operate to establish short, i.e. ten day, courses with special programmes to meet the needs of fieldwork teachers. An unexpected and, in some respects, disturbing feature of this development was the intense interest that the courses aroused among health visitors. In general, large numbers attended who had no expectation of undertaking fieldwork teaching and some employing authorities attempted to send their entire health visitor establishment, a few at a time. This could be interpreted as a greater desire to participate in training, but could also be a response to the nature of courses which, for the first time, had as an objective the identification and study of skills of the health visitor rather than the traditional series of lectures on a range of current topics.

The result may be taken as illustrating the search by many health visitors for a clarification of their function and identification of the skills contributing to their performance. The presence of a number of students with no real expectation of ever working as fieldwork instructors tended to dilute the concentration of the course. However, it is probable that these early efforts contributed to the subsequent work of identifying the particular contribution of the health visitor in the National Health Service and they appear to have been a stimulation and encouragement to many.

ESTABLISHING THE APPROVAL SYSTEM

The appointment of the Joint Secretary in July 1963 enabled a start to be made on an appropriate administrative system for the work of Council, and over the next year the Council established certain Standing Committees.[8] The Education Committee had the task of scrutinising schemes of training and of recommending to the Council whether or not they should be approved. It took a considerable time to find effective methods of appraisal. The relative roles of Council members and professional staff had to be clarified as all were in a learning situation. The training schools also had to deal with the completion of unfamiliar forms. The design of a form which will not impose an intolerable burden on those who have to complete it, yet at the same time gives sufficient information on which to base a judgement is no easy task. Over the years the original forms have been adjusted and modified, a process which is ongoing. The training schools were asked to give details of lecturers participating in the teaching as well as a brief summary of the way in which the various subjects were to be treated. To some extent this would vary among schools according to the resources at their disposal.

The early returns provided an interesting picture of the training schemes. Although most health visitor tutors had attended the teaching course provided by the Royal College of Nursing a certain amount of teaching was carried out by nursing officers without specific training or qualifications in teaching methods. In addition the part played by the Medical Officer of Health could be considerable. On cursory inspection it seemed that the tutor's role was seen as one of organisation, some of it at a fairly humble level, rather than as teaching. In later discussion with colleagues engaged as tutors at that time it seems that this may have been a problem of semantics. Many tutors called their classes and lectures 'tutorials' since they were conducted by tutors, and the early returns of work in the training centres may therefore have been somewhat misleading in these instances.

To some extent the dependence upon medical staff was related to the finance of health visitor training. In most cases the cost was absorbed into the Health Department budget and in some authorities, medical officers of health indicated to new members of staff that their duties would include lectures in the health visitor course. This can be compared with nurse training. Until the Nurses Act of 1949 nursing service and education had come from the same pocket. With the establishment of Area Nurse Training Committees for general nursing, that pocket, i.e. the National Health Service, was subdivided. In view of the long history of containing the cost of training within the Health Service budget it is not surprising that health visitor courses were placed in the same position. Matters had been improved somewhat for basic training with an extension of the authority of the General Nursing Council in 1949 to design an overall budget and to distribute the sum agreed by the Exchequer to the Area Nurse Training Committees. The problem of the health visitor stemmed to some extent from the tripartite nature of the National Health Service, as her service was financed by Local Authorities. The result was that financial responsibility for training the health visitor was being borne by a relatively small number of Health Authorities, i.e. those who chose to operate a training school. Other areas might send students but did not in general make a realistic contribution to the cost, despite the adjustments referred to earlier. There were examples of sharing the burden, for example, the joining of five Local Authorities to finance health visitor training in the South of England,[9] or the provision of two tutors in one university seconded by the city and the adjacent county respectively.

REFERENCES

1 CTHV Training Rules 1965.
2 Bendall, E. R. D. and Raybould, E. *History of the General Nursing Council of England and Wales, 1919–1969*, H. K. Lewis 1969.
3 *Handbook for Health Visitor Tutors and Examiners,* CTHV. First published September 1966.
4 *CTHV Proceedings of Council* HV/M/7 (4.11.63).
5 HC Debate (1961–62) 665, c.1697.
  HC Debate (1961–62) 665, c.16.
  HC Debate (1961–62) 665, c.6w.
6 Red Cross and St. John Joint War Organisation (1939–46) and its successor from 1946 onwards, the Joint Committee of the Order of St. John and the British Red Cross. HSA scholarships are still available.
7 England and Wales Rate Support Grant (Health Authorities) Pooling Arrangements 1968, 444.
  Scotland Rate Support Grant (Local Government, Scotland) 1967, 715.
These statutory instruments updated all existing arrangements.
8 For example Education Committee (see Appendices VI and VII(a)). Recruitment Committee.
9 O'Connell, P. E. 'Community and Hospital in University Nurse Education: The Southampton Experience', unpublished thesis, 1976.

Chapter 5

IDENTIFYING THE FUNCTION OF THE HEALTH VISITOR

How can I know what I think till I see what I say.
GRAHAM WALLAS

THE RELEVANCE OF THE WORK SETTING TO THE HEALTH VISITOR'S FUNCTION

The Council's aim of relating training more closely to the actual work of the health visitor has been emphasised in Chapter 3. Although definitions had been given of health visitors these tended to be vague and general. That given by the Jameson Report as the giving of 'Health Education and Social Advice'[1] had little meaning other than for those most closely associated with the service. It did not help the family doctor, now becoming interested in a closer working relationship with the Local Health Authority Nursing Service, to understand the contribution a health visitor might make. The move to associate the health visitor as the family visitor with the general practitioner, i.e. the family doctor, had been encouraged by, for example, statements such as that in 1954 by the British Medical Association and the Society of Medical Officers of Health. Various systems were developed and have been described. One of the early developments was in Oxford[2] which indicated that the emphasis was on relieving the pressures on the general practitioner rather than the more positive identification of the health visitor's contribution. Her nurse background caused considerable confusion; frequently, what was sought by the doctor was a level of work resembling more closely that of junior members of the ward team than of the ward sister organising care. It is unfortunate that there is not, as yet, a generally accepted view of the particular skills of the nurse.[3] Instead a picture is presented of a considerable number of technical procedures which are constantly changing, some being assumed from those originally carried out by doctors and some being transferred to other workers or technicians as being 'non-nursing'. With this background it was not surprising that unreal expectations of the health visitor were aroused.

REPERCUSSIONS OF THE CREATION OF THE COUNCIL FOR TRAINING IN SOCIAL WORK

This lack of a clear and accepted definition of both the nurse and the health visitor causes equal frustration to the hard-pressed general practitioner and the misunderstood health visitor. The advent of training on a more regular basis for social workers as a result of the Health Visitor and Social Work (Training) Act has added to the confusion. In the past health visitors have frequently filled gaps and therefore tended to be thought of as members of the social rather than the nursing services. That this was attractive to some health visitors is not in dispute. The lack of training opportunities other than those for specific forms of social work and often based on previous academic courses resulted in a number of nurses who were drawn to the social aspects of their work, training as health visitors and concentrating in this area. Reference has already been made to the debate on the original Bill in the House of Lords when Lord Newton indicated one of the Council's objectives as 'The forging of links'[4] between the groups. The absence of a joint secretary and the change in joint chairmanship in the early life of the Council somewhat delayed an approach to this aspect of the Council's work. Both Chief Professional Advisers were faced as their first goal with a formidable task in the establishment and/or renewal of training centres. Professional staff did however begin some joint discussion as to how they saw the respective roles of health visitor and social worker.

It was perhaps the problems inherent in attracting students to train which brought home to the health visitor members of the Council and the professional staff the need to give a clearer professional identity to the health visitor and the range of work actually covered. As the only professional worker normally visiting families at home as part of a statutory service the health visitor tended to be deployed to meet a variety of needs, some initiated by the Medical Officer of Health, some by social agencies who required further information on families in their care and a large number by the general public. This was well illustrated at a later date in a study commissioned by the Council for the Training of Health Visitors and carried out by the Greater London Council's Intelligence and Research Unit[5] in which thirty-four topics, many of which could only be said to be peripheral to the health visitor's stated functions, were identified having been introduced in the first instance by families and individuals visited. 'Topics might range from a relatively simple—almost routine—thing like the need for a fire guard at home, to a complicated problem arising from a threat of eviction. Some of the topics covered were essentially medical, such as phenylketonuria, some were essentially social, such as the language difficulties of an immigrant and many were of the in-between category, neither essentially medical nor non-medical but on the awkward boundary where the problems of the person's mental and physical well-being merged into problems of day-to-day living and had to be reviewed in a complex and urban development.'

ESTABLISHMENT OF A JOINT ADVISORY COMMITTEE FOR THE TWO COUNCILS

One of the peculiar difficulties was that the Medical Officer of Health was the responsible officer in the Local Health Authority for the statutory service. Although therefore the individual health visitor was required to exercise considerable initiative in case finding, decision making, and counselling to families visited, she could never assume full responsibility for the design of her service. This may well have been an important factor in delaying both the definition of her contribution and the excision of some of the multifarious, but outmoded, duties which had accumulated over the years. Apart from personal frustration, this might well result, on occasion, in service being duplicated by more than one department. The Council for the Training of Health Visitors was under considerable pressure by medical officers and senior nursing personnel to publish a statement on the function of the health visitor and there was much discussion in its meetings of a statement produced by members and the Chief Professional Adviser. Eventually a memorandum was sent to the Council for Training in Social Work proposing discussions and a Joint Advisory Committee was set up in December 1964[6]. The objective was discussion of two papers : 'The Function of the Health Visitor' prepared by CTHV and 'The Aims and Objectives of the Two Year Courses' prepared by CTSW. Meetings began under the chairmanship of Lord Morris; in all six took place as well as a short residential seminar.

The setting up of the Councils—not directly related to the provision of services—allowed a quality of debate which, if it did not produce a solution, allowed the individual committee members to develop a better understanding of, and sympathy with, the philosophy of their counterparts. There can be value in a degree of conflict, opposition serves to clarify thinking. Discussion was largely unstructured but was initiated by memoranda from professional staff, which described training in both its theoretical and practical aspects.

The Joint Advisory Committee endeavoured to compare and contrast the service of the two workers to the community and they had in mind some of the findings of an international seminar held in 1959 in which this same topic had been considered.[7] Some of the relevant seminar findings were :

(1) Public health nursing and social work were two distinct functions usually performed by two types of worker.
(2) . . . they remained at the core separate and distinct with their own body of knowledge, point of entry, working methods and professional skill.

'Focus on families tended to suggest that social workers were only concerned with crisis or breakdown. This might be true of direct case work services to individual families but it tended to obscure the positive action undertaken by social workers in neighbourhood or group services, and in contributing to planning preventive or remedial action.' In the discussions in the Councils' Joint

Committee it appeared, in a very general sense, that the health visitor had a continuing responsibility for contact with families due to her statutory position, while the social worker's contact could be better described as episodic. The health visiting service therefore provided an ongoing regular assessment of the health of families and individuals while the social services responded to some lack or need either overt or tacit.

REPORT OF THE JOINT ADVISORY COMMITTEE

Difficulties were encountered when the participants proceeded to consider the contribution of training and how specific this should be. The Health Visitor Council had set out a syllabus with five distinct areas while the Social Work Council had been less explicit. There was clearly a division of opinion here, the Health Visitor Council felt that there could be dangers in too general an approach. The Committee completed its discussion by agreeing a report which was presented to both Councils. The recommendations were as follows :

(a) The Councils should plan at least for some time to come on there being two separate workers, the health visitor and the social worker, in the health and welfare services, but that a degree of overlap of functions between the two workers should be welcomed.

(b) The central functions of these two workers should be as stated above, i.e. the health visitor is a nurse and not a social worker, though her service contains an element of social work; the social worker though not a nurse, is involved in her work in the problems of personal health.

(c) The Councils should keep closely in mind developments in the relationships with general practice; . . . and

(d) The Committee should examine further the question of common ground for training.

The Report was not received with marked approval by either Council.[8] It was not to be expected agreement could be reached in a limited time on a subject which had provoked much discussion over many years, but the operation of a Joint Advisory Committee was an extremely useful exercise.

THE CONTROVERSY CREATED BY DEFINING
A HEALTH VISITOR AS A NURSE

For the Health Visitor Council one of the problems in the report was the description of the health visitor as a nurse and it was decided that more thought should be given to this fundamental issue before any further statement was completed. In addition, it did not appear opportune to continue to examine the common ground in training. A small working group of the health visitor members of Council was therefore established. This group met frequently and completed its initial deliberations at a residential seminar in Edinburgh. In view of the protracted discussion which had taken place at Council on this difficult topic it was thought that the service of a non-Council member as chairman would assist progress and the group was greatly helped when Miss E. M. Wearn agreed to act in this capacity. Although from a related field, i.e. district nursing,[9] she was not involved in the health visitor service. She was, however, well known to many through her past chairmanship of the Public Health Section of the Royal College of Nursing (1958–65). The end of the deliberations gave rise to a brief document of two pages.[10]

There had been for many years a fairly clear division in health visiting between those who felt their expertise was a development of nursing and those who felt it was related to, and indeed part of, social work. The reaction to the original Bill of the two principal professional organisations concerned with health visiting has been described in Chapter 1. If health visitors appeared doubtful about their contribution, however, there was no lack of comment and advice from other fields. Writers studying the health service in general were prepared to write and speak about the health visiting service. The use of the word 'nurse' had long been a problem and the Council gave attention to this in their evidence to the Committee on Nursing.[11] Undoubtedly a number of social workers and social scientists, as well as the general public, have deeply stereotyped views of the nurse. Because training begins in hospital she is thought to be rigid and authoritarian. There may be a kernel of truth in all stereotypes and a training in which the student is inevitably at times in the stressful surroundings of pain, disease and death will obviously have great impact upon its students. This is not the place in which to enter upon discussion of whether or not a fairly brief exposure to such an environment will produce unalterable personality traits but repetition of these views in conferences as well as less formal discussions coupled with, for example, articles such as 'The Uncertain Health Visitor'[12] added to the ambivalence of the health visitor's view of her nurse background. Controversy over the triple duty nurse, i.e. carrying out district nursing, midwifery and health visiting duties was longstanding, in general it was a concept strongly supported by, among others, the Queen's Institute of District Nursing.

THE SECOND STATEMENT ON FUNCTION AND TRAINING

It was obvious that further thought must be given to identifying the skills of the nurse so that consideration could be given to the extent to which these were transferable to work outside hospitals where more than technical competence, in the clinical sense was demanded. The next step therefore was an enlargement of the original simple, very general statement and in May 1967 the Council asked that such a group should be established to prepare a more extensive pamphlet.[13]

In order to have a broadly based discussion, the Chief Professional Adviser recommended seeking the help of some non-Council members and a new working group on the function of the health visitor under the chairmanship of a member of Council, Miss J. Tinch was established. In the event, it seemed that some of the impetus of the purely professional group was lost in the second stage and it may well be that the decision to incorporate a much wider expression of opinion was premature. It had been anticipated that the group would publish the findings but the discussions were not conclusive and the pressure of other developments in the working and structure of the Council inhibited progress. Instead, the report of the group was received by the Council and incorporated in its Fourth Report (1969). There proved to be a large demand for this and subsequently the relevant sections were extracted and made available in a small pamphlet.[14]

The statement aroused criticism, it was thought to be too general and too all embracing. It did however stimulate discussion and was an early example of a number of statements on the health visitor by professional bodies, e.g. 'The Future of Public Health Nursing in Relation to the Community' by the Royal College of Nursing, and 'Health Visiting—A Manifesto' by the Health Visitors' Association. It served to emphasise further the very different approach to training adopted by those concerned with the preparation of the student nurse on the one hand and the health visitor on the other. There was neither immediate nor later reaction by the former to the Council's views on the skills of the nurse. Indeed, the Committee on Nursing in its recommendations on training appears to employ the traditional approach of experience in areas of work rather than identification of underlying sciences. The problem created by reliance on a previous training controlled by a separate body with a different philosophy is therefore obvious. It is possible that the establishment of a new central body concerned with all aspects of training as advocated by the Briggs Report may achieve the marriage of these very different partners but this will depend upon the willingness of all the constituent parties to learn from experience.

THE COUNCIL AS AN ADVISORY AND CONSULTATIVE BODY

The work on the identification of function was not confined to a specific working group, there were many occasions when the Council wished to contribute to discussion on the work of the health visitor particularly in relation to her co-operation or contact with other workers. This was done by setting out the new aims in training and discussing the expectations employers and colleagues might have of students. The extent to which such opportunities arose varied. In some cases the presence of a member of Council in a special working group resulted in a personal invitation to the Chief Professional Adviser to meet the Committee concerned, e.g. in 1965

a sub-committee of the Standing Medical Advisory Committee considering Child Welfare Centres under the chairmanship of Sir
Wilfred Sheldon. The Council might be invited to offer its views,
e.g. to the Local Authority Personal Social Services Committee (the
Seebohm Committee) or might take the initiative in submitting
observations, for example, The Child Health Services Review (the
Court Committee) March 1974.

   The apparent inconsistency in the occasions on which the
Council was consulted was possibly a reflection of its unusual
position. Although concerned in preparing members of the profession for a second qualification it was not a professional organisation in the same sense as the Royal College of Nursing or the
Health Visitors' Association. Its members might be proposed by
these bodies but did not attend as delegates, being appointed
because of the particular skill and experience they could offer on
training. Indeed, at an early stage there was some criticism that
the Council, in setting out its views on the health visitor was
usurping the role of the professional organisations. Nevertheless,
no responsible training body can operate efficiently without a clear
picture of the kind of worker it is hoped to produce and, unfortunately, this picture did not exist in 1962. The debate which
stemmed from the effort to crystallise thinking on training objectives inevitably produced more clearly defined views and it may be
regretted that more consistent use was not made of the thought
which underlay the Council's policy. The publication of the
Council's Second Report (1965) drew an encouraging comment
from *The Medical Officer*.[15] 'This report forms an impressive
justification of the need for the institution of the Council for the
Training of Health Visitors. It has already created some order out
of what was becoming a chaos of training schemes and is turning
its attention increasingly to the big questions about function and
demand that so urgently need answering if enough good recruits
for health visiting are to be obtained.'

THE HEALTH VISITOR AND
GENERAL MEDICAL PRACTICE

One of the areas in which both function and demand were creating
concern was that of health visitors in the family doctor practices.

The city of Oxford had begun associating a health visitor with general practice in 1956, (see p. 47) and its Medical Officer of Health writing in December 1962 stated its objectives as being to assist the general practitioner and to extend the 'catchment' area of the health visitor. The practice was followed in a number of areas and in a report of the Department of Health and Social Security reference was made to the number of staff 'attached' by that time.[16] The subject therefore had great topical interest. The concept of the delivery of care being made by a team was gaining ground and it formed the background for a number of conferences to which family doctors, district nurses and health visitors all contributed. None of these gatherings expected to reach a conclusion on exactly what the word 'team' implied, but there was debate on what the membership should be and, what was perhaps the more emotive question, of who should be its leader. There was a growing awareness of the need to consider the work of the health visitor in relation to other colleagues and this was reflected in the Council's views on training.

In the absence of a clear definition of a nationally accepted description of the health visitor's function, however, it was inevitable that her contribution to the service varied from a complete involvement and use of her contact with all age groups for the initiation of health education, to a very limited and somewhat tenuous contact related to laying on of welfare services. This was an extravagant use of her skills and served only to distract from the other work in maternity and child welfare which she was expected to continue outside the lists of any single general practitioner.

The Council, therefore, had to give much consideration to the expanded work opportunity which attachment to general practice might give, to ensure that training matched this opportunity and to outline for the benefit of employers and colleagues what the aims of the course were. The Council offered information on training and the rationale upon which it was based to the sub-committee of the Standing Medical Advisory Committee under the chairmanship of Dr Harvard Davis in 1969.[17] In this, emphasis was placed on her contact with a more extensive range of vulnerable groups than the traditional mother and child and the associated health education. A further example of the Council's effort to clarify the work which the health visitor trained in the new system might do was the joint pamphlet prepared by the Scottish Advisory Committee of the Council along with the Scottish Council of the Royal College of General Practitioners on the health visitor in general practice.[18]

This need to identify the health visitors' function underlay much of the Council's work, particularly in the years 1963–67.

The same theme can be traced in its discussion with other organisations and in the research projects which it commissioned or with which it was associated. Many of the difficulties the Council encountered in the attempts at definition are related to the large body of health visiting staff trained in an old syllabus and working in a 'pedestrian' (in every sense of the word) and limited environment. The refresher courses which many had attended had not in the past specifically considered health visitor skills but had rather provided series of lectures on single topics.

Selection of candidates for training had been poor in some areas and many medical and nursing officers had set their sights too low in the expectations they formed of potential students. A pessimistic attitude had developed and possibly the journalist writing on the first report of the Council was indicating a more widespread unease : 'We are encouraged by the general farseeing and confident attitude of the Council on the future of health visiting—a refreshing contrast to the apparently pessimistic attitude of the General Medical Council over the Medical wing of the Public Health Service.'[19]

This description of the Council's activities in identifying the function of the health visitor indicates that its role in practice is not so clear cut as the Act would suggest. There is a considerable degree of overlap between a statutory body concerned with training and the professional organisations and the need this creates for good communications will be considered further in the next chapter. It can be seen that the role of a statutory body in relation to the profession it serves merits much more discussion. The Council, however, felt justified in its proposals and took steps to see that these became widely known through its publications and by means of its contact with other interested bodies.

REFERENCES

1 *An Inquiry into Health Visiting* (Jameson Report), HMSO 1956, para. 293.
2 Warin, J. F. *The Medical Officer* (7.12.62).
3 Two attempts at definition are now widely accepted:
   (1) 'The unique function of the nurse is to assist the individual, sick or well, in the performance of those activities contributing to health or its recovery (or to peaceful death) that he would perform unaided if he had the necessary strength, will or knowledge. And to do this in such a way as to help him gain independence as rapidly as possible.' (Henderson, V. *Basic Principles of Nursing Care*, International Council of Nurses. Revised edn. 1969, p. 4).
   (2) 'The nurse is a person who has completed a programme of basic nursing education and is qualified and authorised in her country to supply the most responsible service of a nursing nature for the promotion of health, the prevention of illness and the care of the sick.' (International Council of Nurses, 1965).
4 HL Debate (1961–62) 240, c.1123.
5 Marris, T. *The Work of the Health Visitor in London. A Survey 1969*, Greater London Research Department of Planning and Transportation Research Report No. 12 G.L.C. July 1971.
6 *CTHV Proceedings of Council* HV/M/15 (9.11.64).
7 UN/WHO *The Role of Health Workers and Social Workers in Meeting Family Needs*, Report of European Seminar 1959.
8 *CTHV Proceedings of Council* HV/M/24 (19.5.66).
9 Miss Wearn was employed by Surrey County Council as Superintendent of the Home Nursing and Midwifery Services. In 1966 she became a Public Health Nursing Officer at the Ministry of Health.
10 CTHV *The Function of the Health Visitor*, 1967.
11 CTHV *Evidence to the Committee on Nursing*, 1970, paras 19 and 20.
12 Jeffreys, M. 'The Uncertain Health Visitor' *New Society* (28.10.65).
13 *CTHV Proceedings of Council* HV/M/30 (18.5.67).
14 CTHV *The Function of the Health Visitor*—Implications for Training.
15 *The Medical Officer*. Editorial (21.10.66).
16 Abei, R. A. *Nursing Attachments to General Practice*, HMSO 1969.
17 *CETHV Proceedings of Council* HV/M/49 (13.1.72).
18 CETHV and RCGP (Scottish Council) Joint Report 1973.
19 *The Medical Officer*. Editorial (8.10.65).

Chapter 6

FINDING THE STUDENTS

How beautiful the Emperor's new clothes are.
What a splendid train and they fit to perfection. . . .
'But he has got nothing on' said a little child.
The Emperor's New Clothes—HANS ANDERSEN

The establishment of the first new statutory body with responsibility in nursing since the creation of the General Nursing Council in 1919 aroused little interest in the main body of the profession—a fact commented on in an editorial of the *Nursing Mirror* in December 1961. Health visitor training however was based upon general training and with the few exceptions of the integrated SRN/HV courses (see Chapter 7) all candidates were already registered nurses. It was important, therefore, to establish good communications with the other statutory bodies and the professional organisations in order to improve recruitment to courses and to facilitate discussion of the base upon which the Council had to build. The problem of poor recruitment to training was one of those highlighted at the first Council meeting (see Chapter 2). The members did not wish to emulate the Emperor of the fairy story by providing a new and stimulating training to which no students came nor to make claims for the contribution of a health visiting service which had no members.

LACK OF PRECISE DATA ON CANDIDATES

For some time the Standing Conference of Health Visitor Training Centres had drawn up an annual list of numbers accepted for training and a less precise statement of places unfilled at the beginning of the academic year. This latter list was of limited value as many of the training schools worked to a variable class size and numbers would fluctuate according to local conditions. It was difficult, therefore, to discover how many candidates were refused as unsuitable, how many because the school of their first choice was full and of this latter number how many did not seek a vacancy elsewhere. The Council, exercising its power under the Act, 'seeking to attract suitable persons to training', established a Committee to consider the many facets of the problem. It had been noted by staff that in many instances candidates refused vacancies were not given advice on future action. In part this may have been due to a system in which candidates applied to a future employer for financial support. The interviewing panel would, therefore, be considering the applicant as a member of staff in that particular locality. The fact that she might not appear suitable for some work settings did not necessarily mean that she was not an appropriate candidate for training.

VARIATION IN ESTIMATES OF STAFF ESTABLISHMENTS

There was no central guidance to Local Authorities on the number of staff required to provide an adequate health visiting service as part of a planned development. Figures had been published giving average numbers in post and recommending a goal to which Local Authorities might work, i.e. 0.17 per 1000 population.[1] In the past some authorities estimated the required number of staff on the number of births in an area, others on the overall size of the population. Yet again some estimated on the numbers of children under five and at school.

There had long been a tendency to prefer candidates for training to be over twenty-five years as it was felt they had acquired professional confidence. It is not possible to enter into a long discussion about the value or otherwise of years alone to a potential student but one effect of this policy, sometimes overlooked, was that with the slow development of new training places, staff who had entered prior to the Second World War were now looking forward to retirement. According to a questionnaire sent to Local

Authorities by the Council in 1963, 2093 full time and 385 part time health visitors were between 50 and 60 years of age and therefore likely to retire during the succeeding 10 years.[2] Council staff found in discussion that a number of authorities had no consistent policy of training candidates in advance of known retirements in staff. In Scotland this was even more complex because the Health Visitor Certificate was not obligatory there and a statutory instrument requiring certification was not introduced until 1965.[3] Many of the Local Health Authorities operated a triple duty service, i.e. the one nurse was health visitor, district nurse and district midwife. In 1963, out of 940 nurses so employed, two-thirds did not have a Health Visitor Certificate.[4] These authorities were, in many cases, affiliated to the Queen's Institute of District Nursing and they tended to rely upon that body to produce candidates from its Central School of District Nursing and did not attempt to recruit their own staff. The position in Scotland in relation to numbers of staff not in possession of Health Visitor Certificates was therefore a cause of considerable anxiety to the Council.

It was not easy to obtain a clear picture of the number of health visitors in post in the country as a whole. The growth of health visiting from the maternity and child welfare service and the subsequent deployment of many health visitors in the education service in addition meant that two Government Departments were involved. The Department of Health published figures of whole time health visitors operating in the services for which it was responsible with a second figure of part-time staff also concerned with another service, i.e. mainly the education service. This was frequently misinterpreted. If the Council was to set realistic goals in relation to recruitment it was necessary to obtain further and more precise information about practising health visitors. Accordingly a questionnaire was distributed to the health authorities and the results indicated the size of the task. To assist those health authorities with low establishment to reach the recommended average for England and Wales would require an increase from 650 places to 1072 annually.[5] Increases were also required in Scotland and Northern Ireland. The expansion in numbers did not take account of the increasing tasks allocated to the health visitor (sometimes without consideration of whether or not they were appropriate to her skill but simply because she was there). It was not within the Council's powers to define how the health visitor should be deployed, it could only set out the knowledge it was hoped to impart and to develop. In setting the early goals for student intake the Council was well aware the task was just beginning. It was decided to concentrate on two groups, the newly qualified nurses and those who had left the profession after training.

METHODS OF REACHING POTENTIAL STUDENTS

Since the number of student nurses in training greatly outnumbered the trained staff in the training hospitals, it was obvious that there must be a considerable pool of State Registered Nurses in the United Kingdom who for one reason or another did not proceed to a post in the hospital service. Many married on completing training and did not maintain contact with the profession. As health visiting offers an opportunity to those who are able to bring knowledge from a nursing background as well as experience of married life and a family the Council was anxious to reach such possible recruits. Quite apart from their maturity, such candidates, possessing a settled home in an area, could contribute an element of stability to any staff.

In order to reach both groups in a businesslike way the advice of the Department of Health and Social Security was sought and as a result contact with a firm of advertising consultants was established. The first obvious need was for informative and attractive leaflets of a general nature outlining training, its content, costs and job opportunities. One of the professional staff had particular responsibility for this area of the Council's task and, together with the consultants, a series of leaflets was produced, at first mainly directed at the nurse nearing the completion of training. Great care was taken that all the illustrative material showed actual health visitors in some of their day-to-day activities. The Council was most fortunate in the co-operation given by several health authorities in London. Suitable health visitors as models were suggested, and facilities for photographing given with great willingness. The leaflets were supplied on request to Local Health Authorities and are still in demand by their successors, the Area Health Authorities and Health Districts.

The leaflets were of value when special efforts were being made in specific areas. To ensure they reached young nurses generally was more difficult. In these early years of the Council's life, the degree of general career guidance given to the student nurse appeared to be non-existent in many instances, although a number of training schools were appointing career advisers. These posts varied in scope however, a point upon which the Council commented in evidence to the Committee on Nursing.[6] Too often it seemed to a weary health visitor tutor sifting through applications for the health visitor course that the main criteria for recommending health visiting as a form of work was some physical disability in the student or some failure in her practical ability as a nurse. An approach by the Chief Professional Adviser to the then Hospital Matrons' Association for discussion produced no response. Possibly, it was a naïve expectation at a time when the objective in recruiting the student nurse was the provision of immediate staff in hospitals.

DISPLAYS AT EXHIBITIONS

At that period there was a long established annual nursing exhibition and conference organised by the *Nursing Mirror* in London. It was decided to rent a stand and this became an annual event until the journal changed its policy and the exhibition was discontinued. Once more the Council was indebted to the employing London authorities for their support. Each was invited to supply staff to man the stand on a rota basis and the current 'model' on the leaflet was there on the opening day. This meant that questions would be answered by health visitors in practice and the whole project had a sense of reality and immediacy. As the exercise was repeated and as other consultants became involved over the years the staff developed considerable expertise in deploying their limited resources.

The annual exhibit proved a most useful 'shop window'. In 1969 nearly 1200 enquiries were dealt with during the exhibition and London Boroughs had about sixty enquiries immediately following the event.

THE COUNCIL'S FIRST FILM

The last item in the appeal to the student nurse was the design of a film. It must be remembered that the Council did not have access to unlimited funds and the film is another example of the informal co-operation already described. In this case, in the course of a routine visit to a college, contact was made with a lecturer who had already made some short documentary films. He was interested in the Council's work and accepted a commission from the Council to design a film based on actual students and health visitors. Once more there was a willing response from the authorities approached for co-operation. This time the setting was the industrial North-West and a lively and attractive film *Quite an Education* marked the Council's first experience in this new medium. The film was made on a very low budget and therefore the technical resources were limited. Nevertheless this first effort was received enthusiastically on its preview on 6 November 1970 when it was shown to an audience representative of nursing and medical organisations and press, along with Council members.[7] It has been in constant demand ever since and additional copies have had to be provided.

ENCOURAGING THE MATURE CANDIDATE

An appeal to the older woman was the next stage in the Council's efforts. The report, *Marriage and Nursing* in 1967[8] indicated some of the problems associated with encouraging a return to nursing after a break of a number of years. Despite what might have been thought to be an attraction, i.e. a working day more easily fitted to family commitments, the proportion of married women who had chosen some form of work in the Local Authority service was less than expected. In 1950 60 per cent of married women were in nursing outside the hospital service and of those nursing in 1959 this figure was even smaller, i.e. approximately one-third. Personal communication from one of the research organisers indicated that a number of the nurses expressed interest in work in the community but had little knowledge of its scope and availability. It was recognised that the regular insertion of an advertisement in a nursing journal, one of the methods used to inform the student nurse, was unlikely to reach this wider audience. In many cases the nurse leaving her profession to marry would have become involved in family matters and no longer be reading professional journals. It was necessary to reawaken interest in a return to the profession and to its health visiting section. This had a number of aspects, for example, ensuring that in any 'back to nursing' drive the special attraction of health visiting was included, mounting the Council's own recruitment drives in selected areas and more general efforts to interest journalists, television and radio personnel in the work of the nurse in the community. As these developments involved much time and the learning of new skills, the Council's staff was increased in 1968 to allow one professional adviser to devote the greater part of her time to this activity.

In promoting recruitment the Council worked closely with Local Health Authorities and colleges where courses were planned or were already in operation and a recruitment drive was very often a precursor to a new course. The colleges would supply the accommodation and, with the Council's staff, speakers for the main session. The Local Health Authorities would supply nursing officers to discuss with those interested the prospects in their individual areas and volunteers to come and look after any pre-school children brought to the main session while the Council acted as the general initiator, co-ordinator and supplier of literature.

The success of the first film emboldened the Council to attempt a second *Live and Learn*. This time the appeal was to the older candidate and particularly the married woman. The setting for this film was a Midlands city; once more only real situations were chosen. The main figure was a married woman and the film followed her progress in the first term of the course.

Both films have proved extremely useful and have had a secondary and unforeseen effect. The first, in particular, was in great demand by schools of nursing and it was apparent that it was being used as a description of the work of the health visitor. The films were not designed with this end in view and did not attempt to give a complete picutre. They were designed as a vehicle of recruitment and the aspects shown were those thought to be attractive to the age group concerned. This indicates a need for more thinking on teaching this aspect of nursing in pre-registration courses and raises questions which cannot be debated in this account of the aims and objectives of this part of the general nursing syllabus.

DISCUSSION ON A CENTRAL CLEARING HOUSE FOR APPLICATIONS

After an initial drop in intake, the policy of the Council appears to have been successful and the graph (Appendix III) shows the gradual rise in the numbers of candidates entering training. The issue of two circulars[9] in 1972 from the Government Departments greatly assisted the upward trend by indicating norms towards which health authorities should strive. These recommended a ratio of health visitor staff to population of around 1:3000 or 4000 which would entail considerable expansion of existing establishments. The Council, therefore, carried out a small study to see if there was a substantial number of would-be health visitors refused vacancies either because of shortage of places or because they did not appear suitable. If so it might be desirable to establish a central clearing house.

A continuing cause for concern was the lack of agreement on occasion between training schools and employing authorities on what constituted desirable attributes in candidates for training. Some nursing officers feared that potential recruits were lost to the service because they did not conform to an ideal dear to the training school and if refused at one training school such applicants did not always seek vacancies elsewhere. Equally, some training schools were under great pressure in areas of shortage to accept candidates whom they felt would neither contribute fully to the course nor find a happy and fulfilling job in the future. It was thought that processing of all applications at a central source might overcome these difficulties and in addition ensure a more even distribution of candidates over the country.

Although in the study extending over one year, the position regarding candidates refused a first application did not indicate the need for any clearing house, problems were still apparent of over-application in some schools with vacancies remaining in others. In 1968 the Council staff offered a service to both schools and enquirers. At the beginning of May each year training schools were invited to inform the Council of the number of places still available and applicants unable to obtain a vacancy at the school of their first choice were advised where application might now be made. The scheme was of help in providing a more even distribution of places. The training schools did not welcome the possibility of a clearing house. The proposal was in general greeted with doubt and suspicion and an assumption that the central body would in some way control the selection methods of individual institutions. In view of the introduction of the UCCA system operating for undergraduates applying to universities, this view was somewhat unexpected. Although no central point for application was, therefore, established, the possibility has been raised on a number of occasions since then.

OBSTETRIC NURSING COURSES AND THE MATURE CANDIDATE

The encouragement of older candidates was not a simple matter of specially designed literature, advertisement and campaign. Training required knowledge and experience gained from previous courses in midwifery or obstetric nursing. Many of the older candidates, however, had not proceeded to midwifery training and had not had an opportunity of experience in obstetric nursing during general training. It was necessary, therefore, to consider how this gap might be filled. In many cases family commitments prevented the potential students from following a full midwifery or Part I midwifery course and the necessity for a period of night duty added to their difficulties. Discussions were instituted early in the Council's life with the Central Midwives' Board for England and Wales and it was accepted that candidates could take part in courses approved for student nurses. In order to ease the financial burden in those hospitals willing to accept such pupils it was agreed that as the preparatory course was essentially part of health visitor training the pupils could be sponsored and therefore paid by the Local Health Authority responsible for the remainder of the course and a circular explaining this was issued by the Council. Facilities in Scotland were different. In 1964 a four week obstetric nurse placement for all students training there for the general part of the Register was introduced. The Council did not consider this an adequate basis for the health visitor course and discussions took place with the Central Midwives' Board for Scotland on an extension which would be available to those candidates already accepted for a health visitor course. A circular on this was sent to Local Health Authorities on 24 December 1968 (H & W Services Memo 43/1968).

RECRUITMENT OF STUDENTS AND THE ROLE OF CTHV

The responsibility to attract students to training is one of the many differences between the Council and the other statutory bodies, i.e. the General Nursing Councils and Central Midwives' Boards. In its evidence to the Committee on Nursing, the Council suggested that it is the proper responsibility of a training body.[10] Health authorities may still feel strongly that as future employers responsibility for recruitment and therefore selection must lie with them, but there are dangers in relying too much on either of the partners in the process of preparing future health visitors. One Local Health Authority nursing officer taking part for the first time in the selection of a group of candidates, not all from her own area, regarded her nominees somewhat ruefully when she saw them in the context of others and remarked that her swans had turned to geese. On the other hand, training schools, still jealously guarding their independence can well become detached from the real situations and too readily discard potentially sound and mature students. The Council's advice to the training schools at the time was that interview boards in schools should include a representative from an adjacent authority on a rota basis and that she should see a mixture of candidates, not all seeking future employment in her area. While common goals in selection must be established between service and education, there would seem to be a good case for including a responsibility to the attraction of recruits in the duties of any central training body. It is in their syllabus that clear statements of the general requirements for training can be set out and the general prospects for the future professional development of the candidates and specific employment outlined.

RELATIONSHIPS BETWEEN THE STATUTORY BODIES

This chapter began with a description of one aspect of the Council's activities in what might be best classified as 'communications'. Reference has already been made to the involvement of Council staff in publicising training. There was also a great need to establish relationships with the other statutory bodies concerned with nursing and midwifery; it was, after all, upon their training programmes that the post-certificate health visitor syllabus rested. The Council was greatly encouraged by an early approach from the Secretary of the Central Midwives' Board in London inviting the Chief Professional Adviser and the Joint Secretary to visit and talk about matters of mutual interest. Further visits took place to the General Nursing Council for England and Wales and the professional organisations and similar arrangements were made in Scotland and Northern Ireland. Considerable goodwill was engendered between the officers of the various training bodies, but although there was easy and informal consultation there was need for a more systematic joint effort.

Under the Act[11] the two General Nursing Councils were consulted on two appointments to the Health Visitor Training Council although there was no reciprocal arrangement for the Council for the Training of Health Visitors to nominate members to the General Nursing Councils at that time.[12] As the representatives concerned attended in a personal capacity there was no regular reporting in either direction. Approaches were made by the Council for the Training of Health Visitors to the General Nursing Councils to establish a regular contact and some meetings took place. These, however, served to demonstrate the difficulty of finding a common ground. The Council's goals of training and the methods by which these were to be achieved differed so greatly from those of the other bodies that it would have been unreasonable to expect that progress could be achieved except after a considerable time. This relationship between health visiting and nursing has occupied many discussion sessions over the years.

The suggestion had been made in 1962 that the Council for the Training of Health Visitors might be linked with the General Nursing Council (see Chapter 1). This development was prevented not merely by the fact that with more than one General Nursing Council in existence the United Kingdom concept of the new body would have been impossible, but as early as 1946 the Standing Conference of Health Visitor Training Centres had established a subcommittee to study the training of tutors. Early in their deliberations, its members considered a proposal for a course with a common core for sister tutors and health visitor tutors. This was eventually rejected as it was feared that the large component of the physical sciences required by the sister tutors would not allow sufficient teaching input on the behavioural and social sciences required by the health visitor tutors. This lack, therefore, of a common ground, as reported above, was demonstrated well before the inception of the Health Visitor Council.

The lack of a regular reporting system was highlighted when changes were introduced in nurse training which had implications for the authorities already committed to providing fieldwork for health visitor training, e.g. the introduction of an option in 1969 in England in preparation for state registration and a short obligatory period in Scotland in basic training. In each case observation and teaching of community services were required. In 1971 the Northern Ireland Nurses Act gave the Northern Ireland Nurses' and Midwives' Council similar powers of nominating a member to the Health Visitor Council, once more there was no reciprocal arrangement. It would appear therefore that while it was expected that a nurse from the general field might make a contribution to the thinking and planning of one form of post-certificate education, it was not thought that a health visitor Council Member might similarly have a contribution to make to general training through experience in that Council. In many cases the nominee from the Nursing Council to CETHV has been a health visitor which further reduces the possibility of enlarging the experience of their members.

COMMUNICATION WITH HEALTH
AUTHORITIES

The lack of a common language with nurses may have been somewhat unexpected. On the other hand it was realised that the Council would have to explain very clearly and fully its policy and decisions to those Local Health Authorities and their medical and nursing staff who were concerned both in sending students for training and in co-operating in the provision of practical experience. The Chief Professional Adviser was particularly anxious to avoid the image of an 'ivory tower' institution and the best, although the most stressful, way of providing this explanation was by the staff going out to various parts of the country when groups of training schools and the Local Health Authorities associated with the field-work could gather together for discussion. Accommodation was usually provided either by one of the authorities or a college and the meeting to which medical officers and nursing officers as well as tutors were invited usually took place in the afternoon to allow ease of travel. To begin with these meetings were quite unstructured and consisted of a statement by the Chief Professional Adviser of the current policy in progress and an invitation to comment or offer criticism. The early meetings were, perhaps, more memorable for the latter than the former. The very fact, however, that the Council's staff were present—able to accept criticism, take comments back to the appropriate committees and were given an opportunity to ventilate grievances or disquiet—bore fruit and after the first round of such meetings it was possible to move to a much more constructive form. In later development a morning meeting was devoted to discussion on some particular item of the training by the tutors and the lecturers concerned, followed by an afternoon meeting in which two members of professional staff would present a particular development for consideration and then a general debate would follow.

The regional meetings continued over the period under review and gave rise to two subsequent developments. The first was a series of four residential conferences for tutors and nursing officers.[13] George Bernard Shaw's phrase 'Those who can't do—

teach' finds a ready response in many professions and health visiting is no exception. Nurse administrators may regard the standards set by tutor colleagues as impractical and unrealistic. It is not easy to accept that the tutor is more concerned with broad principles which will be applicable in a wide variety of settings, rather than purely local issues. Conversely, tutors can become detached in their academic setting and fail to appreciate the harsh realities of providing service within the constraints operating in the former Local Health Authorities or the revised Health Service. The second development was also of residential conferences designed to give the recently appointed Regional and Area Nursing Officers in England information and an opportunity for discussion on the training of a section of their staff for whom they might, following reorganisation of the Health Service, be responsible for the first time. The initial response was poor. A number of the nursing officers suggested nominating a member of staff who held a Health Visitor Certificate although such an officer would presumably already be knowledgeable. Two factors could have influenced the response : first, the new nurse managers were still beset by the demands of the new organisation, second, the Council provided the programme of speakers, staff and general organisation from its own resources but the travel and subsistence of the participants had to be met by their authorities. Later conferences were supported better as were the day conferences arranged in Scotland, Wales and Northern Ireland.

Efforts were made early to achieve a common approach to training by training schools in the four countries of the UK. It must be remembered that in 1962 different systems had existed in England and Scotland and with this end in view meetings were deliberately arranged in which, for example, representatives from the North of England would meet with Scottish representatives from Edinburgh or those from Northern Ireland would meet with the representatives from the North of England in Liverpool. While it could not be claimed that by such efforts a common purpose was achieved, the meetings undoubtedly contributed greatly to a better understanding of what it was hoped to achieve by the new training and the warm support given to the Council by, for example, the Society of Medical Officers of Health following the publication of the Briggs Report[14] indicated an appreciation of the advances made.

A STRUCTURE FOR CONSULTATION WITH PROFESSIONAL ORGANISATIONS

The third group with whom it was essential to make a constructive relationship was that of the professional organisations, i.e. the Royal College of Nursing, the Health Visitors' Association and the Scottish Health Visitors' Association. Although these bodies were consulted on the membership of the Council their nominees were not delegates and one of the early problems was to achieve agreement on professional standards to this end. The idea of a mixed professional and educational group was attractive in the first instance.

The Jameson Committee's Report had recommended the establishment of an advisory body[15] and although the members had in mind that it would serve a somewhat different statutory body from the Council for the Training of Health Visitors, it was thought that there would be considerable gain in having this additional source of opinion in policy making. In addition, the Standing Conference of Health Visitor Training Centres (see Chapter 1) had been one of the most important instruments for change and improvement in health visitor training in the years 1946–62. Although the original function of the Standing Conference was in many ways altered and indeed diminished by the formation of the specialist Council it was desirable to retain and expand the common forum for discussion which it had provided. During consideration of the establishment of a consultative committee the concept of a more widely representative body was pursued. A meeting which was attended by representatives from medicine, nursing and education could provide an opportunity for giving more knowledge of each other's aims and methods and so promote a better understanding. In 1969 such a committee was formally established and the following organisations were invited to send representatives: the Royal College of Nursing, the Health Visitors' Association, the Scottish Health Visitors' Association, the Society of Medical Officers of Health, the Standing Conference of Health Visitor Training Centres and the Royal College of General Practitioners.

The Chair was taken by the Chairman of the Council and a number of meetings were held. Although there was useful discussion, the idea was not a complete success. Few items for the agenda were submitted by other than the Council and the frequent change in the representatives of the organisations attending did not facilitate ongoing consideration of the more difficult questions from one meeting to another. In particular, the representatives of the Standing Conference were not happy with the arrangement and sought their own special form of communication with the Council. Finally, it had to be borne in mind that the demands now being made upon Council members for attendance at various meetings were beginning to prove extremely onerous. With few exceptions all members were in whole time employment. It was possible to reduce the number of Council meetings to four per annum, but the associated service in committees increased greatly the number of occasions a member might have to travel to London, in itself another expenditure of time. Some reduction in the numbers of Council members on the consultative committees was essential.

Eventually it was decided to set up three special groups with one Council member involved in each who would take the Chair. These were :

(1) The Professional Organisations Consultative Committee with representatives of the Royal College of Nursing, the Health Visitors' Association and the Scottish Health Visitors' Association and the Society of Nurse Managers (formerly Society of Chief Nursing Officers).

(2) The Liaison Committee with representatives of the Society of Medical Officers of Health (later the Society of Community Medicine) and the Royal College of General Practioners (and from 1975 representatives from nursing management). Representatives from the related bodies in Scotland were included.

(3) The Standing Conference Contact Group whose representatives were the Chairman and the Honorary Secretary with representatives from each of the regions in which local meetings were organised.

Looking back it would seem that a multidisciplinary group as originally conceived was premature. The experience was similar to that described in Chapter 5 in relation to the expanded working group discussing the function of the health visitor. The venture served to underline the danger of assuming that bringing together representatives of different vocations would of itself produce a common aim and language.

CONTACT WITH THE NURSING DIVISION OF THE DEPARTMENT OF HEALTH AND SOCIAL SECURITY

Reference has already been made in Chapter 2 to the need to establish relationships with the Government Departments. There was no direct membership of the Council – nursing officers and civil servants attended only as Assessors. The Joint Secretary formed his own lines of communication with his administrative colleagues in the various sections of the Departments. It was essential that the professional staff in their turn should have a continuing dialogue with colleagues in the nursing division. In addition therefore to those occasions on which a meeting was arranged by the Department to discuss some proposal put forward by the Council at which administrative and professional staff of both bodies were represented, a series of quarterly meetings was organised with the nursing division. These were intended to provide an exchange of views and a consideration of common problems. This arrangement referred to England and Wales only. The small staff involved in the Scottish Home and Health Department and the Ministry of Health in Northern Ireland made communication simpler and more immediate.

REFERENCES

1 Health and Welfare *The Development of Community Care*, HMSO 1963 Cmnd. 1973. Also *An Inquiry into Health Visiting* (Jameson Report) HMSO 1956. 'We have suggested principles on which the workload could be uniformly assessed by each authority. According to our estimates . . . a total force of 11,500 whole-time health visitors might be

necessary. This should be the approximate target representing an increase of 3,500 whole-time health visitors.' (paragraphs 387–397)

2 CTHV *Proceedings of Recruitment Committee* HV/RC/67/2 (19.1.67) and Appendices.
3 SI 1965 No. 1490 (S.80). National Health Service, Scotland.
4 CTHV *Proceedings of Scottish Advisory Committee* CTHV/SAC/M3 (10.6.63).
5 CTHV *Proceedings of Recruitment Committee* HV/RC/67/2 (19.1.67) and Appendices.
6 CTHV *Evidence to the Committee on Nursing*, para 64, 1970.
7 This and the second film were awarded a certificate of commendation for use in medical education by the British Life Assurance Trust for Health Education with the British Medical Association.
8 Ramsden, G. and Skeet, M. *Marriage and Nursing*. 5th Report of Dan Mason Nursing Research Committee of National Florence Nightingale Memorial Foundation, 1967.
9 DHSS HM (72) 13.
SHHD SHM (72) 10.
10 CTHV *Evidence to the Committee on Nursing*, December 1970, para. 10F.
11 Health Visiting and Social Work (Training) Act 1962. First Schedule 5(c).
12 A change in the constitution of the General Nursing Council for England and Wales gave this facility to the CTHV at a later date (Nurses Act, 1969).
13 The staff of the Council had been concerned at the lack of agreement between the two in many areas and the actual conflict in a few cases.
14 Comments submitted by the Society to DHSS, January 1973.
15 *An Inquiry into Health Visiting* (Jameson Report), HMSO 1956, para. 374.

Chapter 7

THE NEED FOR RESEARCH

Theories are nets—only he who casts ever catches.
Logic of Scientific Discovery—K. POPPER

The Health Visiting and Social Work (Training) Act gave Council certain powers in research, i.e. Section 2(i)(d). At first sight the use of the word 'training' would seem to indicate some restriction of topics. It is clear, however, that training includes, for instance, subject matter, teaching methods, student selection and the nature and assessment of practical experience. The range of activity included in this section therefore is wide. In July 1964 a group was formed to determine priorities.[1] As the Council had few representatives with a particular interest in and experience of research, it was decided to co-opt members with special expertise to the group. The membership in the first instance and the list of topics thought at the first meeting to be relevant are shown in Appendix (IV). The list itself is an indication of the paucity of actual evidence available upon which decisions might be made for this area of nursing.

PROGRESS WITHIN FINANCIAL AND STAFF CONSTRAINTS

Just as responsibility was laid on the Council to establish and maintain standards of training without accompanying specific financial provision, so with research, no specific provision was made for carrying out any investigation and on each occasion the project had to be considered as an independent item. A major consideration must always be the personnel available for any investigation. The tiny professional staff was fully occupied in stimulating and encouraging new training and contact with existing courses. The Chief Professional Adviser who in the early stages maintained a personal contact with new training schools soon found the administrative content of her work precluded even that and certainly made any active participation in actual research impossible. One solution might have been the establishment of a Joint Research Unit serving both Councils but this was not seriously considered. It seemed too early in the relationship of the two bodies to achieve the satisfactory use of a joint resource of this nature.

There seemed no hope in 1964 of enlarging the Council's professional staff overall although the possibility of a dual appointment to the professional staff, half to the Council and half in employment with an appropriate research organisation or university department was considered. The matter was not put forward to committee, although it would have had the advantage of providing on-the-job training for a health visitor in what was at that time a new activity, as some Council members who were consulted were not happy and colleagues in the Government Department were not optimistic. Potential members of staff with research experience were very few in number. The policy which was finally established was twofold, the commissioning of research by appropriate bodies on behalf of the Council, for this, financial support had to be obtained from the Government Department, and at the same time certain small internal investigations to be carried out by one of the professional staff. The cost of the latter had to be met within the overall budget. Although the Council always included a sum in its estimates specifically for research—this was never accepted by the Government Department in approving the budget.

THE GREATER LONDON COUNCIL'S STUDY OF HEALTH VISITORS' RANGE OF WORK

Reference has already been made in Chapter 5 to the Council's early difficulties in identifying the actual work of the health visitor. An investigation in 1950 by the Nuffield Foundation had not been published and the findings of the Jameson Committee were based on work prior to 1956. Change had been rapid in the ensuing years. Contact was established with a university department where a number of investigations on the delivery of health care in the community had been undertaken and a preliminary proposal was discussed at a meeting of the Research Committee. Unfortunately the Government Department did not feel able to support the idea and it was not pursued in its original form. The concept, however, was not dropped and through the help and guidance of a Council member it was possible to interest the Greater London Council's Intelligence and Research Unit, in carrying out a study on the work of health visitors in the thirty-two London boroughs.[2] Although it is freely admitted that London is not typical of the country as a whole, the study with its tripartite base of inner, middle and outer boroughs provided information on varied work settings with which comparisons could be made : for example, with a decayed city centre; some of our great urban developments; with industrial towns and, lastly, with the suburbs surrounding these.

THE NURSING TEAM IN GENERAL MEDICAL PRACTICE

Perhaps the most significant development taking place in the working conditions of the health visitor was her growing association with the family doctor to which reference has already been made in Chapter 5. It was therefore thought desirable to examine to what extent existing courses would fit a health visitor to make a significant contribution and to determine what additional training, if any, would be necessary. To do this effectively the relationship of health visitor and district nurse had to be considered since both were placed in close proximity in this new setting. The part played by the other aides entering the employment of the Local Authorities had also to be examined along with the health visitor's capacity to deploy her new resources. The University of Edinburgh, Nursing Studies Department, was interested in carrying out such a study and a small working group was established to formulate proposals. These were accepted by the Research Committee and submitted to the Department of Health for financial support, and after considerable negotiation these were accepted. The study was of a small team coming together for the first time consisting of health visitors, district nurses, state enrolled nurses, aides and secretary in a practice setting of 12 000 population. The team had a designated co-ordinator, an introductory period on the possibilities of work in the new setting and ongoing counselling during the period of the study which covered one year. Other teams without either previous introduction or ongoing counselling, and in one case no identifiable co-ordinator, were also included as were a number of other teams illustrating a variety of relationships.

A pilot study was carried out and subsequently the main study was published in 1974.[3] There were many difficulties on the way, some due to staff changes during the period of the study both in the University and the Council and the early death of the Director of the University Department involved.[4] There was also difficulty in finding an appropriate area for study. Association of staff with the family doctor had taken place with great rapidity and it was not easy to find a situation in which the study could commence at the beginning with a newly attached nursing team, not previously related professionally either to each other or to a group practice. The Council greatly appreciated the co-operation of doctors, nurses, administrators and above all the 'guinea pig' team in what proved a most useful and interesting study, which points the way to the need for much more investigation in this new field. The impact on training was the not unexpected finding of the Council's Professional Adviser, who acted as the counsellor, that existing courses did not give sufficient background particularly on case-finding or on team relationships to allow health visitors to exploit fully the possibilities of this new arrangement.

The study also served to illustrate again the great dichotomy in training between the ideal and the actual. It was possible to give a classroom picture of the scope of work associated with general medical practice but this had little meaning if the student did not see it carried out. If, on the other hand, training were restricted to those areas in which very good facilities were available, the over-all numbers entering health visiting would never be sufficient to make an impact in the areas where service is limited and unimaginative.

DESCRIPTIVE STUDY OF TWO COURSES OF INTEGRATED SRN/HV TRAINING

In the fifties courses had been developing in some training schools in which a student could become state registered and a health visitor in one integrated course usually within a period of four to five years. The objectives and the nature of the courses varied greatly : in some cases it was hoped to increase the number of entrants to health visiting; in others to make more effective use of the nurse training and, yet again, in some to shorten the overall time required for the various parts of training. The General Nursing Council for England and Wales (no such courses had developed in Scotland) approved the nurse content under the provisions for experimental courses, but no systematic evaluation of the content of courses necessarily followed. Individual courses published reports of their own. The powers under the Act for health visitor training seemed to put the Council in a particularly responsible position to assess progress. In spite of limited resources of staff and equipment there was the pressing need to improve and expand training generally. It was therefore decided to attempt a simple examination of two integrated courses.

The aim was to follow the progress of four groups of integrated course students and to contrast their progress and their reactions with those of other students entering the same institutions but following the orthodox courses. A conspicious difficulty in such evaluations has always been that of comparing like with like. E. Bryden studying the course at Hammersmith had drawn upon candidates of similar educational backgrounds but drawn upon candidates in another training school as the control group.[5] The study the Council had in mind would include a follow through of the intakes of students to the end of the first year after completing the entire training.

It was decided to absorb the cost of the study within the general resources of the Council with the service of additional office help at times of particular activity, for example, the annual return of questionnaires and when other data were being received and collated. Once more the study highlighted the difficulties created by too small a professional staff. With only three professional advisers, absence due to illness, domestic crisis, or a move to another post effectively reduced the resources by one-third, while diversity of other responsibilities diluted the concentration of effort in a particular project. Nevertheless, despite changes in Council staff and the difficulty of maintaining contact with very mobile groups of student nurses, the study was eventually completed, published[6] and is currently under discussion by the Council committees. Although the report is essentially narrative in nature the very problems engendered by the project throw an interesting light on both students' attitude to their training and the type of record maintained of such training.

The General Nursing Council for England and Wales during this time had embarked on a more extensive study of experimental schemes. While the Council's study was under way much discussion had continued on the value and possible future of courses which achieved an integration of health visitor and general nurse training. Courses leading to a university degree either within an established university or within the polytechnic system leading to a degree awarded by the Council for National Academic Awards were being established. The latter, in particular, offered an opportunity to identify the academic base of education designed specifically for nursing and this usually incorporated a substantial component of teaching in the social aspects of health and disease, i.e. part of the health visitor syllabus. Most of the integrated health visitor/SRN courses demanded the equivalent of university entrance in educational qualifications and courses which did not, in addition to a professional certificate, offer the possibility of a degree were likely to be less attractive to candidates. The Council, therefore, had to consider whether there would be a place for the older type of course—already intake to some of these courses had ceased in favour of undergraduate programmes. A further aspect to be borne in mind is whether or not sufficient health visitor content could reasonably be incorporated within a first degree or whether it demands postgraduate work.

STUDY OF THE EXAMINATION SYSTEM BY THE NATIONAL FOUNDATION FOR EDUCATIONAL RESEARCH

This valuable although unpretentious study was an example of the Council's efforts to examine aspects of training which might have been inherited from the previous system and which had implications for future policy. The Council itself had, however, introduced great changes. The introduction of a pattern of such different design to that which had operated previously inevitably produced many problems. Attention has already been drawn to the very varied resources available to each training school. It was decided therefore to establish a working group of the Education Committee to review the syllabus and examination in the light of three years experience.[7] The eventual report which was issued eighteen months later concluded that the design of training was fundamentally sound but some reduction and greater flexibility was introduced into the examination.

The Working Party depended upon observation made by tutors, staff, examiners and students. Such evidence was obviously highly subjective and the Council felt the need to see to what extent, if any, a common standard was being reached. Such an investigation was obviously beyond the resources of the Council's staff. In addition it was desirable that the Council itself should not be involved in such an inquiry if a truly objective report were to be achieved. An approach was therefore made to The National Foundation for Educational Research, their proposed design was accepted by the Research Committee of the Council and the Department of Health and Social Security was asked to assist by making the necessary funds available.

The study required much co-operation from training schools and initially there was considerable doubt about the purpose of the inquiry. In addition to the fears some tutors appeared to have that there was a subtle move back to a centralisation of examination, the nature of the design necessitated much additional work. Both the Chief Professional Adviser and the member of professional staff now responsible for the Council's research interests devoted much time to explanation of the need for the study and its general method, both to individual institutions and to the Standing Conference of Health Visitor Training Centres. To some extent the attitude within the schools was a reflection of the growing desire for autonomy in the various training establishments and was not merely confined to relations with the Health Visitor Council.

The study has now been published[8] and is under consideration by the Council and its committees. Among the findings, those which indicate great variation in standards will be under particular scrutiny. To what extent this variation is due to the Council's system or to the growing pains of learning to operate a different form of assessment it is not possible to say at this stage. The Council's concept of one examiner serving more than one school and then moving after a period of three years to others, so gradually introducing a common measure in the examination, has not proved practicable. It is difficult to find examiners willing and able to give time to a very demanding task and many feel that they must restrict their service to one training school. The annual examiners' meeting although helpful can only hope to provide a forum for discussion on one aspect of examining as well as consideration of the previous academic year's progress.

FIELDWORK: THE RANGE OF EXPERIENCE

The inquiry by the staff into the operation of the two integrated courses was an example of a small investigation which forms part of the responsibilities of the professional staff. Another example is a more recent study made on the availability of various types of practical experience and of the possibility of ensuring a reasonable coverage by the grouping of fieldwork teachers.[9] One of the interesting developments it foreshadows is a consideration of the fieldwork teacher and her place in both service and education spheres.

REFERENCES

1 *CTHV Proceedings of Council* HV/M/13 (27.7.64).
2 Marris, T. *The Work of the Health Visitor in London. A Survey 1969*, Greater London Research Department of Planning and Transportation Research Report No. 12, GLC July 1971.

3 Gilmore, M., Bruce, N., Hunt, M. *The Work of the Nursing Team in General Practice*, CETHV, 1974.

4 Miss Elsie Stephenson, MA, SRN, SCM, SRFN, HV (Cert.).

5 Bryden, E. C. M. *An Integrated Course of Nurse Education: A Study of an Experiment*, Queen's Institute of District Nursing, 1969.

6 Williams, H. M. *Report on the Evaluation of Integrated Nurse Health Visitor Schemes of Training Undertaken by Professional Staff at the Council for the Education and Training of Health Visitors*, 1966–74. CETHV 1976.

7 *CTHV Proceedings of Education Committee EC/68/16.*

8 Fader, W. *Qualifying Experience for Health Visitors*, NFER 085633 1112 1976.

9 *Report on Findings of a Small Investigation Carried out on Fieldwork Range of Experience*, CETHV, 1975. Ref. 1460.

Chapter 8

WORKING TOWARDS A FAVOURABLE CLIMATE FOR DEVELOPMENT

Here lies the body of Henry Day
Who died defending his right of way
He was right, dead right, as he marched along
He's just as dead as if he were wrong.

ANON

One of the outstanding features of the Council's record has been its emphasis on efforts to create a climate of opinion in which the nature and quality of training can flourish and expand, it did not wish to join the late Henry Day. Such a climate is as important to the newly qualified member of staff taking up her first appointment as to the student, indeed subsequent professional development may well be influenced by early experience in post. The various lines of communication which the Council established with related organisations were described in Chapter 6. Here we are concerned with a further step, i.e. the provision of short courses and conferences. It was not clear from the Act just what significance could belong to the phrase 'the further training of health visitors'.[1] The first use of powers under the section related to the provision of courses for fieldwork teachers and the development of courses for this group is described in Chapter 4.

THE COUNCIL'S CONCERN IN MANAGEMENT COURSES

The whole area of courses for senior health visitors in other positions was largely unexplored in 1962. The National Hospital Nursing Staff Committee responsible for a very large-scale operation to provide management training for the nurse in hospital following publication of the report of the Committee on Senior Nursing Staff Structure (the Salmon Committee) in 1966 did not, in the first instance, cover the needs of senior staff in the community. The provision of suitable management courses for this group had great importance for the Council. The training of the health visitor required supervision in the final period by a first level nursing officer : not only were these few in number, fewer still had had any preparation for this work. Here the Council encountered an important barrier to an effective development of its work, probably quite unforeseen when the Act was drafted, i.e. the Council's responsibilities referred to the training of health visitors only. A majority of nursing officers were responsible for other services, e.g. district nursing and midwifery and the Council, therefore, had no powers to embark upon any plans for the establishment of management courses for such workers. A Departmental Committee, however, was established under the chairmanship of Mr L. Mayston, to study the needs for nursing management in the Local Authority and to compare it with the recommendations of the Salmon Committee. A report was circulated subsequently and Local Health Authorities began to introduce new structures.[2] Although the Council was willing to act as entrepreneur in the provision of courses for management, in view of its experience in working with varying types of educational establishment, its component of members working in managerial positions and its experience in the syllabus planning, such a move was not encouraged by Government Departments. Also in the light of the increasing volume of other work this particular aspect was not considered further. One short special course, however, was held in Leicester in July 1972 in which special emphasis was given to the responsibility of the first level manager in Local Health Authority

Nursing Service for the teaching element of supervision. As the Council was particularly concerned at the quality of practical work supervision, in the final term of the courses, a short prototype course was organised for group advisers[3] in May 1971 and there-after individual colleges were encouraged to consider mounting these within their own resources.

REFRESHER AND OTHER SHORT COURSES

The Council did not see itself as an actual provider of courses but rather as a body concerned in identifying the need and organising resources to meet that need. Nevertheless, there seemed to be three areas in which there should be more direct involvement: one was the organising and running of a prototype which could be used and developed by individual colleges, an example of which has just been quoted. A second was the participation with other organisations in forms of in-service short courses, some of a multi-disciplinary nature, and a third was the direct provision of study days or short courses associated with new developments. A list of the most important of these may be found in Appendix V. In 1969 the Council was asked by the Department of Health and Social Security to consider the provision of refresher courses for health visitors as part of its responsibility for 'the further training of health visitors'. This is an example of co-operation in the second area quoted above and in view of the magnitude of the task it is worth-while setting out the way in which the Council has developed this responsibility.

A number of institutions represent the interests of health visitors and two in particular, the Royal College of Nursing and the Health Visitors' Association provide educational facilities as part of service offered to members. In 1943 the Nurses' Salaries Committee of the Ministry of Health under the chairmanship of Lord Rushcliffe recommended that health visitors should attend a post-certificate refresher course not less than once in five years. This only applied to England and Wales and although Scotland was, therefore, not covered, a few of the more forward looking authorities recognised the importance of continuing development and arranged for in-service courses. In the intervening years the two organisations cited above were the main providers of refresher courses. There was, however, some variety, e.g. some Local Authorities arranged a series of in-service courses, some of a few days, some a week in length. In most cases the latter were only for the staff of that authority but occasionally two or more authorities would join together to provide an annual course to which participants from other areas might be invited. The degree of choice open to a health visitor varied widely. In some authorities she was given no option and might be restricted to courses organised by her employing authority. No common standard was established and no systematic evaluation of the content and quality of the courses offered was made, although the fees and costs represented a considerable outlay for the employing authorities.

The Council staff estimated that if each health visitor attended once in five years there would be a considerable shortfall in the places available when the Council assumed this task. In order to extend the availability of places, colleges interested in joining the scheme were invited to attend a meeting with the two professional organisations. The situation was complex. Each of the professional bodies had established its own design of course over the years. Any proposal that either should not continue to offer courses, or that these should be standardised, would interfere between the body and its members and would be unacceptable. In 1972, Council staff met representatives from the two organisations and three representatives from interested colleges, under the chairmanship of a Council member. Involvement of tutorial staff from the training schools presented a useful development which it was hoped would have a double effect. It was important that tutors should have a continued contact with experienced health visitors in actual practice and to spend a week together in residence would give opportunity for much informal exchange of views and information with which to maintain a practical element in teaching. In addition, courses could usually be provided more economically where some resources were already available.

CRITERIA UPON WHICH TO BASE ASSESSMENT OF REFRESHER COURSES

Agreement had to be reached on a general policy to be pursued on the design of courses, the number of places to be offered in each case, and above all on a system of evaluation. The following paragraphs are taken from the reports of the discussions with course organisers and set out the Council's policy. First it was necessary to define what was meant by refresher course.

It is a planned programme of studies organised on a national basis for practising staff. It is built upon new knowledge and recent developments of practice pertinent to the professional sphere of activity. The objectives are to enable the participant to reappraise, reaffirm and extend a professional level of activity in order to maintain and advance standards. It allows opportunity for the interchange of ideas, the revitalisation of interest, and the consideration of new concepts of work. The course should thus advance professional standards and so promote a more efficient service to the community.

It was important to distinguish between in-service and refresher courses. In-service training should be the responsibility of the employing authority and in particular be related to new skills and service developments in the area. Refresher courses should aim to deal with professional and health service developments in a wider context and provide a forum for an exchange of ideas and experience. Courses should conform to some basic criteria, e.g. as to length. It was agreed that five days would be the most appropriate and the Council was not prepared to accept shorter courses as coming within this general category. The numbers attending should also conform to some pattern. Forty to sixty was considered a desirable number which could produce a variety of experience and ideas and might also be economically viable, there were disadvantages in much larger numbers. Some organisations had in the past accepted applications from different categories of staff. General refresher courses should be for health visitors only, because of the background knowledge and experience upon which the course would be founded. The multidisciplinary courses, which had great value, would, for the present, be in addition to the main provisions.

Over the years the various bodies engaged in refresher courses had developed their own systems of organisation but as much of the success of the course depended upon the overall co-ordination and planning, this should in future be in the hands of one person, a member of the profession (i.e. not a committee), although advice on content might well be obtained from such a source. Most courses were divided into smaller groups working with tutorial guidance and the Council considered there should be a tutor/student ratio of 1 : 20 with the majority of tutors having a health visitor background. The word 'tutor' was used in the sense of adviser and did not imply restriction to qualified health visitor tutors, the object was to provide some degree of counselling with regard to professional development where appropriate. In addition to the course organiser and the tutors there must be clerical and administrative assistance to deal with the general management so that the tutors might have time for the professional side of the organisation.

The Council would also expect a reasonable geographical distribution throughout the year. In the past, there had occasionally been a surplus of places, especially during academic vacations when residential accommodation became available. Courses should provide for residence with adequate rooms for discussion groups but the Council agreed that a small number of participants might be accepted from the locality, provided they did not form more than one-third of the total.

Systematic and ongoing evaluation was essential and agreement was reached on an appropriate form to be returned by those attending the courses. The processing of the information obtained was carried out by the Council staff and the results discussed at the annual study day.

Each of these criteria presented problems. The Council saw the disadvantages of very large course numbers but such courses were cheaper to run and the professional organisations had to cover costs. In some areas accommodation for more effective—i.e. smaller —numbers, was difficult to find. The Council appreciated the great benefit to be obtained from residential courses but the increasing number of health visitors with home commitments and the higher cost to the employing authority could make such courses unpopular.

STUDY DAYS FOR COURSE ORGANISERS

After considerable discussion, a scheme was established by which the number of places provided would be agreed annually, participants would be asked to complete an appraisal form and the Council would circulate to all health authorities information on dates, topics and venue of all the courses which conformed to the agreed criteria. In 1973 the Council arranged a study day on a topic having a bearing on the comments made by the health visitors on the evaluation forms. The first study day concentrated on the place and organisation of group work, frequently the object of adverse criticism by the respondents. Later, this study day was attached to the annual meeting at which the numbers of places and the main themes to be explored were determined.

MULTIDISCIPLINARY COURSES, CO-OPERATION WITH THE ROYAL COLLEGE OF GENERAL PRACTITIONERS

Another example of involvement in actual courses in co-operation with other bodies is what became known to the Council as the 'Windsor Course'. In 1971 the Royal College of General Practitioners approached the Council and the National Institute for Social Work Training to seek their participation in a course for general practitioners, social workers and health visitors. The overall co-ordination was carried out by the Royal College and each of the three bodies co-operated by providing a tutor who would be resident during the four day course.

The experience proved a most rewarding one for tutors and students. Numbers attending were restricted, partly to ensure small enough sub-groups and partly because available accommodation was limited. Employing authorities were invited to nominate students and were asked to choose the recently qualified, i.e. within two years of certificate or degree. In this way it was hoped to reach those still possessed of the enthusiasm of original training and not yet daunted by a possibly restricted environment. The course was described in the *Journal of the Royal College of General Practitioners*[4] and has been the stimulus for further development, the latest being a course for the teachers in the practical setting.

Similar developments took place in study days for fieldwork teachers and tutors. Unfortunately, just as no money was available centrally for the training of tutors, so none was available for any of the above activities. A fee to cover costs had therefore to be set and this affected to some extent the numbers who could attend. Despite these difficulties, however, the Council continued to use this system of gradually raising the standards by agreement and examples of courses and conferences over the years are shown in Appendix V.

THE IMPLICATION OF ACCEPTANCE OF MEN IN HEALTH VISITING

This chapter describes some of the special courses arranged to help qualified health visitors maintain and develop the standards set in their original training. It is a convenient point at which to examine the problem of a group of staff in some health authorities who had been seconded to health visitor training but who had not been able to obtain the certificate at the end of the course—the men. There were two obstacles : the first, related to the wording of the regulation defining health visitors, and the second, to the required obstetric nurse component upon which part of the health visitor course is built.

In the original regulation the health visitor was described as 'a woman' who carried out certain duties. Quite apart from any discussion on the rights or wrongs of restricting entry to any vocation purely on the grounds of the sex of the applicant, the profession was divided on the desirability of including men in this section of nursing. Some health visitors and medical officers could see areas in which health education and counselling might be more acceptable from a man than a woman, e.g. work with adolescent boys in the school service, some work with the elderly and in those families with problems in which it was more than usually important to develop a contact and work with the father. On the other hand if the policy that the health visitor was one of the last of the generalists was to be pursued, it would not be possible to select for some parts only of her work and there might be difficulties in the more traditional work with mothers and young children. Here the public might expect that the unsolicited offer of service and advice would be made by a woman.

An additional factor to be borne in mind when looking on this dispute was the lack of clarity on the specialist as well as general contribution of health visitor and social worker (see Chapter 5). Prior to the Local Authorities Social Services Act (1970), many Medical Officers of Health had responsibility for the welfare services in their authority. It was not unexpected that a number felt communication could be easier with nurses whose training and background was familiar than with the newly emerging social workers. Faced with the need to provide service, e.g. in the field of mental health, encouragement of male nurses with psychiatric training seemed sensible. When the question of a suitable preparation was raised, administrators turned to the existing health visitor courses. Some training schools began to admit men and a number of Local Health Authorities advertised for 'male health visiting officers'. Usually a second qualification was demanded such as Registered Mental Nurse.[5]

The claims of the male health visitor were advanced in many quarters, e.g. a session was devoted to a debate on his contribution to the service at the Annual Congress of The Royal Society of Health in Blackpool in 1966 and an item appeared frequently on the agenda of the Scottish Advisory Committee of the Council. The training school in Aberdeen had been the first to provide training facilities. Early in its existence the Council considered the matter and concluded 'there is a place for men in a good health visiting service bearing in mind the unique contribution they can make in certain fields'. This opinion was forwarded to Government Departments and the matter rested there for some years although it made periodic returns to public discussion.

It is perhaps unfortunate that the Council was pressed for a decision at such an early stage. The conclusion reached then represented rather an acceptance of the *status quo* than a complete consideration of what the training of a male health visitor would entail. With more mature examination of the subject and the experience of the new syllabus, the real significance of the obstetric nursing or midwifery qualification as a prerequisite to the health visitor course emerged. In the former training system a considerable amount of teaching on the prenatal development of the child, the antenatal care of the mother and the immediate consequences of childbirth had been repeated in many health visitor courses. With the introduction of a new and academically more demanding syllabus, this was not possible and reliance had to be placed, quite properly, on the prerequisite qualifications stated in the Council's Rules. It was now clear that the obstetric nursing precursor to the health visitor course was not merely an additional certificate but an integral part of the preparation of the health visitor. In 1966 the Council made its first statement on the function of the health visitor. This implied a worker with a general, not a specialist function. If men were to gain the statutory certificate they would have to carry out the same duties and consequently have the same background and training as their women colleagues; midwifery and obstetric nursing was not then open to the male nurse.[6]

OBSTETRIC NURSING APPRECIATION COURSES FOR MEN

A small working group was convened which included a representative from midwifery and a male nursing officer who had followed the health visitor course and subsequently worked as a health visitor in a large city on general duties. The group discussed how training might be provided should the defining regulation be amended. Two needs had to be met: courses for men already in employment in the health visiting service and who had followed a health visitor course, and courses for candidates accepted for training.

The group identified the objectives of a suitable obstetric nursing appreciation course as giving a firm basis of knowledge on

(i) the prenatal factors affecting the growth and development of the child;

(ii) the emotional and physical factors affecting the mother, baby and family during pregnancy and childbirth;

(iii) the processes of a normal labour and puerperium;

(iv) the special problems of the newborn infant and of the neonatal period.

A plan for observation was devised which included the writing by the student of a study of an 'expectant couple' in which the husband's contribution as well as the well-being of the mother and child were considered.

The regulations were altered in 1972 and 1973[7] to define the health visitor as a 'person' and plans could then be formed for introductory courses.

After much discussion two courses were arranged, each based on a health visitor training school but with very full co-operation from an adjacent midwifery school. One course was in Scotland, one in the London area. The men were well received in the midwifery schools both by staff and those patients they met in the departments. The studies of the expectant parents were particularly successful and provided encouraging views of ways in which an imaginative and constructive service would develop.

Despite the hopes of some of the protagonists for the entry of men the numbers entering training have not made a significant impact on recruitment. Their arrival did, however, have two effects: first, it made the Council members and staff clarify their ideas about the significance of the obstetric nurse component. The second effect is still unresolved. If men can obtain this essential background in a short, specially organised course, why do the women have to undertake the standard placement? The debate continues.

PROVISION FOR UNCERTIFICATED STAFF IN SCOTLAND

Scotland had special needs in relation to short courses. The absence of refresher courses on a regular basis meant that many senior staff had not been given an opportunity of updating. The Council staff therefore organised two short residential courses in

St Andrews for county nursing officers and superintendent health visitors. These provided an outline of the new health visitor training and set this in the context of developments in the health service and in education. The major concern was the large number of nurses undertaking health visitor duties without training. Once the regulation[8] was introduced which made the certificate essential unless dispensation was granted by the Central Government Department, a determined effort was required to overcome the problem.

The Scottish Advisory Committee of the Council established a small working group which in addition to discussion of possible solutions, made two visits to areas with particular problems. Any attempt to provide training for all the existing staff in post was clearly impractical. It was not reasonable to expect that older women, long detached from study, should return to a demanding whole time course. There were also many nurses whose commitment to elderly or dependent relatives would make a long absence from home impossible. The employers, too, would be in difficulty. Many of the areas served by the nurses were remote and not necessarily attractive to temporary staff who would have to be recruited to fill the gap while the individual nurse was on a year's study leave. It was decided to adopt a three part scheme :

(a) A two week orientation course would be organised each year for the older nurse.

(b) A specially designed course (see Chapter 3) for nurses already in post who for family reasons would find it difficult to leave home for more than one term, or for whom the employer would find it difficult to find a replacement.

(c) Every encouragement would be given to young applicants for triple duty work to obtain all the necessary certificates before entering this field of work.

The short orientation courses were organised originally by the Queen's Institute of District Nursing in Scotland in consultation with the Council. The Institute was a familiar body and it was felt that this joint approach would assist the nurses attending to feel more at home with the new ideas. The Council was indebted to the

Institute for co-operating in this new activity. Subsequently, however, responsibility was assumed by the Council staff until the new Health Visitor Training Centre in Dundee was sufficiently established to take this over.

REFERENCES

1 Section 2 (i) (b).
2 *Report of Working Party on Management Structure in the Local Authority Nursing Services,* 1969. Department of Health and Social Security, Scottish Home and Health Department, Welsh Office.
3 This title, first used in the Jameson Report 1956, was used in many authorities to indicate the first supervisory level in the health visiting service.
4 *Journal of the Royal College of General Practitioners,* Vol 22, pp. 603–609, 1972.
5 *First Report of Council for Training of Health Visitors,* 1962–64.
6 Midwives Act 1951. 14 and 15 Geo. 6, Ch. 53.
7 The NHS (Qualifications of Health Visitors) Regulations 1972. SI 1972. No. 1822.
   The NHS (Qualifications of Health Visitors) (Scotland) Regulations 1973. SI 1973. No. 63.
8 National Health Service Scotland. SI 1965. No. 1490 (S.80).

Chapter 9

CONCLUSION

There is nothing permanent except change.

HERACLITUS

The Council's life between 1962 and 1975 as recorded here does not present a picture of unruffled serenity. It may be that in later years it could be said that too much was attempted with very limited resources. Life was reminiscent of the country dance routine, advance, retire and set to partners. The Chief Professional Adviser, as she was originally called[1] was much concerned, however, at the length of the period since the Jameson Report—six years—and the rapid development in the associated field of social work. This concern was shared by members of successive Councils who supported the many innovations. Apart from the ferment of new ideas arising within the Council, the climate in which it had to operate was one of turbulence and change. Out of the many new developments we can select ten reports or changes in legislation which had an effect either directly or indirectly on the Council and its communications. These are:

Reorganisation of Local Government in London	
(Local Government Act 1963)	1965
Senior Nursing Staff Structure (the Salmon Report)	1966
The Related Report on Staff in the Community	
(the Mayston Report)	1969
Post-Certificate Education and Training of Nurses	
Standing Nursing Advisory Committee	1966
Establishment of Joint Board of Clinical Nursing Studies	1970
Social Work in the Community Report	
Scottish Office (Cmnd 3065)	1966

Of these, the three marked with an asterisk had the most pro-
found effect. Reorganisation of Local Government in London and
nine years later in the country as a whole, created problems of
communication and necessitated the establishment of new relationships. They were, however, of greater significance to the service staff
with whom the Council had to work than to the staff of that body
directly. The same might be said of the reorganisation of the
management structure within nursing. To some extent the move
towards a nursing officer with responsibility for the three sections
of service in the community diluted the health visiting expertise in
the most senior position and foreshadowed the results of the greater
reorganisation of the National Health Service and some of the
conclusions of the Briggs Committee.

RESOURCES IN 1970:
CTHV'S PROFESSIONAL STAFF

Before embarking on a consideration of the three items selected for
further discussion we should examine the resources of the Council
by 1970. The initial size of the professional staff of the Council had
placed a heavy burden on those in post at a time when it was particularly important that they should be out and about in the training colleges and the areas of field work. A further problem in a
small staff is the limited opportunity for the stimulus and interplay
of opinion between members of staff. There were also obvious
difficulties in the Council's case in providing for continued staff
development through release to attend courses and conferences.
Efforts were made to overcome this by means of staff seminars to

which research workers in related fields, members of the Council's Research Committee and observers from the Nursing Division of the Department of Health and Social Security, were invited. These were organised three to four times per annum. While it is now accepted that a programme of continuing professional education should be provided for staff in post in many vocations, it would seem that more thought has yet to be given to the needs of those in central positions concerned with the administration of training such as the Council. Although efforts were made to provide for some form of sabbatical leave at regular intervals in the budget this was never achieved. Nevertheless, there was a gradual general increase in staff as a result of a number of negotiations.

INTERNAL REORGANISATION AND CHANGE

The years 1965–70 saw considerable change in the internal and domestic organisation of the Council. Under the Act members are appointed for a period of three years and may be invited by the Secretary of State to continue for a further term. Four[2] of the original Council remained for three terms but the majority served for two. The term of the Chairman is five years. Due to the need to preserve continuity over a time of very considerable reconstruction within the Social Work Council, the Privy Council invited Lord Morris to continue after his term and he remained until 1970. The first Joint Secretary left to take another appointment in 1966 and was succeeded by Mr F. E. Frayn, CBE. As the work was continuing to expand there was much to be done in the design of an administrative structure to support this increased volume for both Councils.

In those years the Council was involved in submission of evidence to many of the committees which foreshadowed the organisational change and it early became obvious that the relationship between the two Councils would alter. This would have implications for the Health Visitor Council in both a policy making and more domestic sense. There is a slight difference in the constitution of the two Councils, i.e. it is possible for the function of the Social Work Council to be extended to 'other social work' (Section 3 (3) Health Visitor and Social Work (Training) Act 1962). There was no similar provision for the Health Visitor Council. The effect, therefore, of the Social Work Order of 1971[3] was to be an expansion of the Social Work Council which would immediately create an imbalance between two bodies which had begun life as equal partners and which shared common resources.

SEPARATION OF THE CHAIRMANSHIP OF THE COUNCILS

The first effect was a separation of the chairmanship. It had been hoped that by setting up two organisations under one Chairman and having some members in common that some joint goals might be established (see Chapter 1 and Appendix VI). In practice the idea proved impractical. The proliferation of standing committees as the Council's business grew, as well as the necessary full meetings required by both bodies, could involve a joint member in at least two or three visits to London every month. The principle therefore of common membership came under strain before 1970 and although both organisations had been particularly fortunate in having as Chairman Lord Morris, who was prepared to give considerable time to the affairs of both Councils, his term of office was ending and it would not be easy to find one person willing and able to give the necessary time. The division of office of chairman was therefore inevitable. Professor W. J. H. Butterfield, OBE, DM, FRCP at that time Vice-Chancellor of the University of Nottingham accepted office for the Health Visitor Council. His colleague on the Social Work Council was Sir Derman Christopherson, Vice-Chancellor of the University of Durham.

IMPLICATIONS OF ENLARGED RESPONSIBILITIES OF THE CENTRAL COUNCIL FOR EDUCATION AND TRAINING IN SOCIAL WORK

The consequences of development within social work in advance of the reorganisation of both the National Health Service and Local Government have been the subject of study and comment elsewhere and this book does not set out to identify the main course of

subsequent events. Simply from the point of view of the Health
Visitor Council, it was peculiarly unfortunate that decisions had to
be taken relating to the expansion of the Social Work Council
while the report of the Briggs Committee was awaited (which
would certainly affect the position of all the statutory nursing
bodies). An additional difficulty was created in that many of the
Council members were deeply involved in the reorganisation of
their own service in the health authorities. They could be facing
not merely a change in the scope of work but even the disappearance of actual positions such as that of Medical Officer of Health.

In many respects the Councils had never functioned as joint
bodies. There was some interchange between professional staff but
efforts to achieve a common policy in respect, for example, of
courses in those colleges where training for both certificates was
being carried out in the same department were unproductive. By
1970, the number of professional staff for the Social Work Council
had already grown to twenty-eight and in a period of uncertainty
and stress there was much to be gained if each Council could have
its own chairman.

Absorbed in the reorganisation of the National Health Service
it is possible that the immediate effects of the reorganisation of the
Social Work Service as proposed by the Seebohm Committee may
have been obscured for leaders in medicine and nursing. The
immediate impact on the professional staff of the Council was the
realisation that the health visitor in the field upon whom the training colleges and consequently the Council had to rely for practical
work teaching was, in many areas, unsure of the future. Council
staff found themselves frequently called upon for reassurance as
representatives of an organisation outside the actual service.

The revised Social Work Council, now known as the Central
Council for Education and Training in Social Work,[4] grew out of
the nucleus of the original Council for Training in Social Work
but due to the need to marry the diverse training bodies which now
came within its ambit there was a strong desire to establish it as a
new body and to dissolve the relationships arising out of the past
system of work. The tenuous link therefore between the social
work and health visitor professional staff was more and more
eroded and it became obvious that this would have implications for

the joint administrative staff. The move towards complete separation came closer.

Discussion of what might be required to sustain a separate Health Visitor Council was hampered by the need to await the outcome of the Briggs Report which did not appear until 1972 as well as the reorganisation of the National Health Service. The two Councils continued in the same office block where additional accommodation was acquired and there was an expansion of the joint administrative and office staff to serve both Councils. This enlargement could only be regarded as a temporary expedient while awaiting further discussion on the future of both bodies.

Well aware that even more far reaching changes than those facing the Social Work Council could be expected, in view of the sheer magnitude of the reorganisation of the National Health Service as a whole and of nursing in particular, special thought was given to relationships with other nurse training bodies. In addition to the continued informal contact between officers of the various statutory bodies there were two others with whom the Council could be closely associated. One was the Panel of Assessors set up by the Secretary of State in relation to district nursing training. Attention has already been drawn (Chapter 5) to the overlap in the work of social worker and health visitor, equally important was the overlap in the work of health visitor and district nurse.

HEALTH VISITOR AND DISTRICT NURSE TRAINING

The increasing association of Local Health Authority staff with the family doctor has indicated the need for some clarification. The decision of the General Nursing Council for Scotland in 1967 to include a period of observation in the community as part of a comprehensive training and the resolve of the General Nursing Council of England and Wales to offer an option in this aspect of nursing in 1969 emphasised this further. It might have been desirable to have put district nurse and health visitor training under the direction of one statutory Council at an earlier date but there was considerable resistance to this by the respective professional

organisations. Nevertheless the Royal College of Nursing submitted its views to the Government Department[5] on the need for
a unified approach to the training of nurses in the community.
In the debate on the Local Authority Social Services Bill a proposal
that this might be achieved by a similar method to that used for
the Social Work Council, i.e. by means of an amendment to the
Training Act was put forward by the opposition but was rejected.
In speaking on this, however, Mrs Shirley Williams replying to the
proposal[6] indicated that while it would be wise to await the report
of the Briggs Committee; 'it would be our intention during the
next few years to bring the Panel of Assessors and the training
coming under it as closely as possible in touch with the Council
for the Education and Training of Health Visitors and the Central
Council for Training in Social Work with a view to seeing what
steps should be taken in the light of the Report of the Briggs Committee'. No action, was taken by the Government Department but
the Council, in consultation with the Panel, was able to establish
a committee with members from both parties chaired by the Chairman of the Panel, Mr Robson, the administrative and secretarial
support being provided by the Council. The meetings did not make
any significant progress and were discontinued at the request of
the members of the Panel of Assessors. It was hoped that the
situation would be clarified by the Briggs Committee and the
Council referred to the matter in its evidence to that body.[7]

THE JOINT BOARD OF CLINICAL
NURSING STUDIES

The other new body was the Joint Board of Clinical Nursing
Studies, originally set up in March 1970 to advise on the post-
certificate clinical training of nurses and midwives in special departments of the hospital service and to co-ordinate and supervise
courses provided as a result of such advice. In April 1973 the
remit was extended by the Secretaries of State for Social Services
and for Wales to introduce responsibility for nurses and midwives
in specialist aspects of the community services in England and
Wales. As this was at a time when more far reaching changes could
be expected as a result of the deliberations of the Briggs Com-

mittee, this may well have been precipitate and presented a contrast to the caution over district nurse training. It introduced yet another confusing factor into a situation in which two bodies already had responsibilities, one by statute, i.e. the Health Visitor Council, and the other with a specific responsibility set up by the Secretary of State, i.e. the Panel of Assessors.

Early in the life of the Board, the Chairman of the Council had invited Sir Hedley Atkins, then its Chairman, and Miss Gardener, its Director, to meet with him and the Director of Education and Training for discussion, and helpful informal contacts were developed. Acting on the principle that the best way of achieving understanding was to undertake a joint project, steps were taken to include a clinical content for health visitors in some refresher courses. Despite the good relationship, however, there were problems in the consideration of courses impinging on the health visitor/district nurse field such as preparation for the practice nurse and others.

THE REPORT OF THE COMMITTEE ON NURSING

The Briggs Report was published in 1972 and was greeted with very mixed feelings. Considerable hostility was expressed by the organisations representing health visiting and the Council viewed a number of the proposals with concern.[8] These were mainly concerned with the establishment of single vocational training institutions outside the mainstream of education, the proposed shortening of the health visitor preparation and the dilution of expertise and energy which would follow the delegation of training powers to education boards in each of the three countries, England, Scotland and Wales. (Ulster was not included in the original remit of the Committee.) This seemed to favour a return to the pre-1962 position in relation to health visitor training. There was also disappointment in some quarters that the Committee had apparently failed to grasp the nettle of the overlap between health visitor and district nurse.

Much discussion lay ahead on the possible implementation of the Report which had many controversial aspects related to other fields of nursing. The future for the Council was therefore still uncertain and during the period 1972–75 the staff had to contend with the obvious change and growth of the Social Work Council and all that this implied in the internal life of both bodies, along with doubts and fears among tutors and field staff and uncertainty on their own future. Despite this very troubled atmosphere, the staff worked with determination and optimism, recruitment of students continued to rise, new training centres were established and new developments such as the extended courses for more mature candidates grew more surely.

SEPARATION OF THE TWO COUNCILS

Pressure was now mounting in the Social Work Council for further separation. Demands on its staff to expand training facilities, to identify priorities and to prepare a programme for advance over a period of years increased so that the Council could regard its immediate future as secure. In January 1973 it decided to seek the separation of the administrative resources of the two Councils. This presented legal problems, e.g. the lease of the premises was held jointly and there was a joint secretarial staff of considerable size. Discussion had to take place, therefore, in the Health Visitor Council which was in a particularly vulnerable position. The Chairman set up a small working party to decide what his Council would require in order to continue to operate with dignity and efficiency for an interim period. The problems were in part domestic, e.g. the division of the existing accommodation and the position of the joint staff but there was also another, less tangible, but equally important, consideration. The morale of health visitors, particularly those associated with training, had suffered a severe blow in the Briggs Report. Many were also apprehensive about the forthcoming changes in the National Health Service. It was important that they should not be made to fear that what many had come to regard as one of the new representative symbols of health visiting, i.e. the Training Council, was being dismissed as relatively unimportant.

Discussion on the nature of arrangements which would secure a stable environment for the Health Visitor Council for an interim period was not easy. Separation of resources would involve the disappearance of some posts and the creation of some new ones. The Health Visitor Council decided on a structure which would have a Director supported by two principal officers, one concerned with administration and one with professional matters. There would be twenty-eight administrative staff and eight professional advisers. The new administrative pattern operated from 1 October 1974 and coincided with the triennial reappointment of the Council (see Appendix VII and Appendix VIII.

REFERENCES

1 The title was changed to Director of Education and Training in 1971.
2 Mr Rule, Joint member; Professor Pemberton; Miss D. J. Lamont; Miss P. E. O'Connell.
3 Central Council for Education and Training in Social Work Order. SI 1971. No. 1241.
4 The original title of the Health Visitor Council was expanded at the same time to Council for the Education and Training of Health Visitors under the terms of the Local Authority Social Service Act 1970 which was brought into force in the UK on 1 October 1971 by SI 1971. No. 1221 (C.31).
5 *Rcn Evidence to the Committee on Nursing*, June 1971. This was followed by Rcn comments on the *Report of the Committee of Nursing* (February) 1973.
6 HC Debate (1969–70) 801, cc. 974, 976.
7 CTHV *Evidence to the Committee on Nursing* (December) 1970, para. 53.
8 CETHV Comments on the *Report of the Committee on Nursing* (February) 1973.

POSTSCRIPT BY THE AUTHOR—1978

The story ends at this point, three years have passed since the decision was taken to separate the resources of the two Councils. It is clear that it has not in any way impeded the progress of the CETHV but the intervening period has raised other questions and an account of these must await some future occasion. Looking back on those exuberant, troubled but constructive twelve years some may regret that what began as an imaginative attempt to achieve an integrated approach to training in both the health and social services did not develop. Rather what emerged was a more clearly identified difference between the two workers, nevertheless this clarification alone is to be welcomed. Many may also regret that the very different but apparently successful training policy of the Council did not commend itself to the Committee on Nursing. This has given rise to apprehension lest the advances achieved between 1962 and 1975 could be lost in a general reshaping of nurse training along with an overenthusiastic attempt to provide that training in a more comprehensive form before the knowledge base of its constituent parts has been identified.

Some uncertainties remain but there are also grounds for encouragement, the most obvious are the achievements in health visitor training but there are certain other developments outside the Council's immediate sphere. It is noticeable that nurse/undergraduate courses developed early in those universities and polytechnics in which there was a nucleus already provided by a health visitor course such as Southampton, Surrey and Manchester while the Polytechnics of Newcastle upon Tyne and the South Bank in London have pioneered the ordinary and honours degrees in nursing within the scope provided by the Council for National Academic Awards. The Council, then, may feel pride in the advances listed in the summary to this chapter and all the other features of a flexible and forward-looking body but may find the greatest ground for optimism in this more subtle influence. The contribution to be made to the base upon which the post-registration courses can be built will be highly significant if the nurse of the future is to receive the preparation which will allow her to change to meet new and emerging needs, and above all to find personal fulfilment in the profession she has chosen to enter.

SUMMARY OF MAIN INNOVATIONS

TRAINING

Syllabus based upon broad areas of study.

New examination pattern with decentralisation and external examiners drawn from a variety of disciplines.

Incorporation of student's study of fieldwork in the examination.

Extension of training to one calendar year.

Inclusion of short period of supervised practice following the academic year.

Training to be in educational institutions with fieldwork in associated health authorities.

All candidates to have the General Certificate in Education in five subjects or an appropriate alternative.

Obstetric nursing appreciation courses for men following the change in regulations.

Assumption of responsibility for the Roll of health visitor tutors.

New facilities for tutor training.

Establishment of courses for fieldwork teachers.

Provision of adequate facilities for refresher and other short courses.

RECRUITMENT TO TRAINING

Design and publication of a range of literature, redesigned annually.

Design and distribution of two films.

Advice and assistance in areas of special difficulty.

Provision of training facilities in new areas.

New forms of training to attract the mature candidate.

Participation in national and local exhibitions.

COMMUNICATION

Joint Advisory Committee with Social Work Council.

The Royal College of General Practitioners on short multidisciplinary courses.

Establishment of consultative machinery with the professional organisations.

Staff co-operation with the other statutory bodies, the Panel of Assessors and the Joint Board of Clinical Nursing Studies.

Regular inter-staff meeting with some members of the nursing division of the Department of Health and Social Security.

Regional meetings at regular intervals with employing authorities and associated training schools.

Residential seminars for tutors and nurse administrators.

Association with the Standing Conference of Health Visitor Training Centres.

Regular news bulletins outlining new developments, changes in policy and giving the background to much of the Council's objectives.

General reports at intervals (five in number).

Selected pamphlets and leaflets : *Function of the Health Visitor;*
Function of the Health Visitor and Implications for Training;
Joint Report by the Council and the Scottish Board of the Royal College of General Practitioners;
Evidence to the Committee on Nursing;
Observations of the Council on the Report of the Committee on Nursing.

Appendix I

MAJOR DEVELOPMENTS IN HEALTH VISITING 1906-1962

Date	(1) Legislative Measures or Reports (2) Major landmarks in Training	Provisions
1906	Huddersfield Corporation Act	Required notification of births within the city.
1907	Notification of Births Act	Notification of births at the discretion of local authorities.
1908	The Royal Sanitary Institute (founded in 1876) Examination for Health Visitors	
	London County Council (General Powers) Act	Empowered sanitary authorities to employ women health visitors.
1909	Health Visitors' (London) Order for London C.C. area	The Local Government Board established the first statutory qualification for health visitors in the London area.
1915	Notification of Births (Extension) Act	Required notification of births within 36 hours (Compulsory for whole country).
1918	Maternity and Child Welfare Act	Established local authority services for expectant and nursing mothers and children under five years on a firm basis.
1919	Board of Education (Health Visitors' Training) Regulations	Established two types of courses : (1) For 2 years for inexperienced students (2) For 1 year for trained nurses or others possessing substantial experience.

Date	(1) Legislative Measures or Reports (2) Major landmarks in Training	Provisions
1919	Scottish Board of Health established. Issued regulations for training and examinations	
1925	Ministry of Health became responsible for the training of health visitors	
	The Royal Sanitary Institute designated the examining body	
1928	Ministry of Health regulation	Full-time officers were required to hold the health visitor's certificate.
1929	Local Government Act Statutory Rules and Orders (1930 No. 69)	Laid down qualifications for health visitors and tuberculosis visitors.
1936	Public Health Act	Repealed previous legislation and laid down new requirements.
1944	Education Act and School Health Service Regulations, 1959, Reg. 5, S.I. No. 363	Every nurse employed by the education authorities for the purpose of the school health service should have the health visitor's certificate.
1946	The National Health Service Act	
1948	The National Health Service (Qualifications of Health Visitors and Tuberculosis Visitors) S.I. 1948 No. 1415	Identified a health visitor as a woman "employed by a local health authority for the visiting of persons in their homes for the purpose of giving advice as to the care of young children, persons suffering from illness, and expectant and nursing mothers, and as to the measures necessary to prevent the spread of infection and also includes a woman so employed by a

Date	(1) Legislative Measures or Reports (2) Major landmarks in Training	Provisions
1948		voluntary organisation under arrangements with a local health authority."
		A 'tuberculosis visitor' "means a woman employed by a local health authority for the visiting of the homes of persons suffering from tuberculosis for the purpose of giving advice as to the care of such persons and as to measures necessary to prevent the spread of infection and also includes a woman so employed by a voluntary organisation under arrangements with a local health authority."
	Establishment of courses for health visitor tutors by Rcn in co-operation with the City of Birmingham Health Department (until 1958)	Thirteen students were accepted – ten had grants from the Ministry of Health and two from the Department of Health for Scotland.
1950	The Royal Society of Health – Revision of Syllabus	Widened the subject matter and altered examination system to allow longer time between written and oral examinations. Written examinations to be held in training school.
1956	An Inquiry into Health Visiting (Jameson Report) HMSO June 1956.	The Report of the Working Party set up in September 1953 under the chairmanship of Sir Wilson Jameson. Produced the most fundamental examination of the work and training of the health visitor to date.
1962	Health Visiting and Social Work (Training) Act The Royal Sanitary Association of Scotland – Revision of Syllabus	Established the Council for the Training of Health Visitors and the Council for Training in Social Work.

COUNCIL FOR THE TRAINING OF HEALTH VISITORS
MEMBERS OF THE FIRST COUNCIL 1962-1965 (APPOINTED IN SEPTEMBER 1962)

Chairman : Sir John Wolfenden, CBE (resigned July 1963)
Sir Charles Morris, KCMG, later Lord Morris of Grasmere, appointed 1 August 1963

(1) The original members of Council appointed in September 1962 :

Miss J. Armstrong, RGN, SCM, HV
Dr J. C. Arthur, OBE, MB, BS, MRCS, LRCP
Miss N. B. Batley, SRN, HV (resigned 18 February 1963)
Councillor Mrs F. E. Cayford, JP (resigned 24 February 1964)
Professor T. E. Chester, MA
Councillor A. Cunningham, JP
Miss M. E. Davies, SRN, SCM, HV
Miss J. Ewart, RGN, SCM, QN, HV
Miss G. M. Francis, SRN, SCM, HV
Alderman N. Garrow, OBE (resigned 5 March 1964)
Miss A. A. Graham, OBE, SRN, SCM, HV (resigned 11 March 1965)
Miss R. Hale, SRN, SCM, HV Dip. Sec.Sc (London), RFN
Miss D. T. Hogg, SRN, SCM, HV
Miss R. A. Hone, BA, SRN, SCM, DN
Dr J. G. Howells, MD, MRCS, LRCP, DPH
Miss D. J. Lamont, SRN, SCM, HV
Dr B. R. Nisbet, OBE, MD, FRCP, DPH
Miss P. E. O'Connell, SRN, HV
Professor J. Pemberton, MD, FRCP, DPH
Mr A. M. Rule, MBE, MA, LL.B
Alderman Mrs Ryder Runton, CBE (resigned 20 March 1963)

Alderman Mrs P. Sheard, BA, JP (resigned 18 November 1963)

Miss J. A. Surr, SRN, SCM, HV

Dr H. P. Tait, MD, DPH, FRCP (resigned 5 May 1965)

Dr E. Thomas, BSC, PhD (resigned 5 September 1963)

Dr W. E. Thomas, BSC, MB, BCh, DPH, MRCS, LRCP

Dr G. W. H. Townsend, CBE, BA, MB, BCh, DPE

Dr J. F. Warin, MB, DPH (resigned 1 March 1963)

Councillor J. R. Watson

Miss E. E. Wilkie, BA, SRN, HV (resigned 16 April 1963)

Professor R. C. Wofinden, MD, DPH, MRCS, LRCP

(2) Changes in membership 1962–64 :

Dr E. L. Millar, MD, DPH, MSC, appointed vice Dr Warin 1 March 1963

Alderman A. H. Davies, appointed vice Mrs Ryder Runton 20 March 1963

Miss A. L. Adair, SRN, SCM, HV, appointed 26 August 1963 vice Miss Batley and Miss Wilkie

Mrs E. Beith, SRN, HV, appointed 26 August 1963 vice Miss Batley and Miss Wilkie

Mr R. E. Hodd, BSC (ECON), appointed 16 January 1964 vice Dr E. Thomas

Mr C. Berridge, appointed 4 March 1964 vice Alderman Garrow

Councillor K. C. Collis, appointed 3 December 1964 vice Mrs Sheard

Appendix III

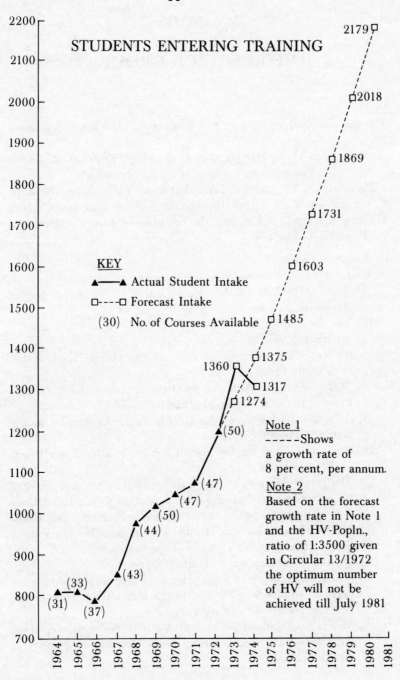

STUDENTS ENTERING TRAINING

KEY

▲——▲ Actual Student Intake

□----□ Forecast Intake

(30) No. of Courses Available

Note 1
----Shows
a growth rate of
8 per cent, per annum.

Note 2
Based on the forecast
growth rate in Note 1
and the HV-Popln.,
ratio of 1:3500 given
in Circular 13/1972
the optimum number
of HV will not be
achieved till July 1981

Appendix IV

THE RESEARCH GROUP

The first informal meeting of this group took place on 9 November 1964.

Present: Miss M. E. Davies, Miss D. T. Hogg, Professor Wofinden. Dr Townsend sent apologies for his absence.

The group had to consider first, what topics came within the scope of the Section 2 (i) (d) of the Health Visiting and Social Work Training Act 1962, and second, the co-option of further members to the Research Committee.

1. *Research Topics*

   Under this heading a number of suggestions were made:

   (1) The contribution of the Health Visitor to the Local Health Authority services.

   (2) The Health Visitor in liaison with the General Practitioner
       (a) what duties does she carry out
       (b) what 'image' does the General Practitioner have of the Health Visitor.

       (Reference was made to research already carried out by Pinsent, Backett, Shaw and others.)

   (3) A large-scale survey of the Health Visitor in relation to the National Health Service.

   (4) The contribution of the Health Visitor in after-care schemes for Mental Health.

   (5) The Health Visitor's changing role in relation to other workers, for example, her changing role in relation to the Child Care work with the neglected child (Child Life Protection Act 1963).

   (6) Job satisfaction for the Health Visitor, does her work after qualification measure up to her expectations?

   (7) Quality of supervision of Health Visiting work.

   (8) Consumer reaction to the Health Visitor. (Reference was made to studies by PEP and to the indirect reference in the Newsom studies in Nottingham.)

   (9) Methods of individual Health Visiting, for example, what criteria does the Health Visitor use in determining priority in Health Visiting?

Appendix V

COURSES AND CONFERENCES

The professional staff of the Council contributed to a large number of conferences and courses organised by training schools or professional bodies over the years. It is not possible to itemise all such occasions but the following is a list of activities for which the Council was directly responsible or in which the staff undertook a substantial amount of teaching. With few exceptions all were residential.

Most were designed to introduce the new syllabus or new aspects of training and, after an initial period, responsibility for some was assumed by training schools.

Courses varying in length between 2 and 10 days

Fieldwork Teachers (Scotland)	2
Senior Local Health Authority Nursing Staff (Scotland)	2
Triple Duty Nurses without Health Visitor Certificate (Scotland)	3 or 4
Group Advisers	1
Health Visitor Tutors	4

Courses in participation with other organisations

Fieldwork Teachers with University of Glasgow Extramural Department	1
Triple Duty Nurses (original orientation courses) with Queen's Institute of District Nursing (Scotland)	2
Group Advisers and Nursing Officers with Polytechnic of Leicester School of Management	1
Social Workers, Health Visitors, General Practitioners promoted by Royal College of General Practitioners and with the National Institute for Social Work Training	2

Study days

Health Visitor Tutors (prior to establishment of annual courses)	4

Refresher Course Organisers	3
Tutors to Fieldwork Teacher Courses	3

Conferences

Regional meetings with Health Visitor Tutors and
    Local Health Authority Nursing and Medical Senior
    staff
    2 to 3 per annum   Total 30 approx.

Residential Seminars for Superintendent Nursing
    Officers and Health Visitor Tutors before 1974   4

Residential Seminars for Health Visitor Tutors and
    Regional and Area Nursing Officers following
    integration of the National Health Service   3

Residential Conferences for Council Members

Workshop for Health Visitor Members only   1

Symposium for Council Members and Guests
    'Towards Integration'   1

Appendix VI

COUNCIL STRUCTURE 1970 (SHOWING RELATIONSHIP WITH CTSW)

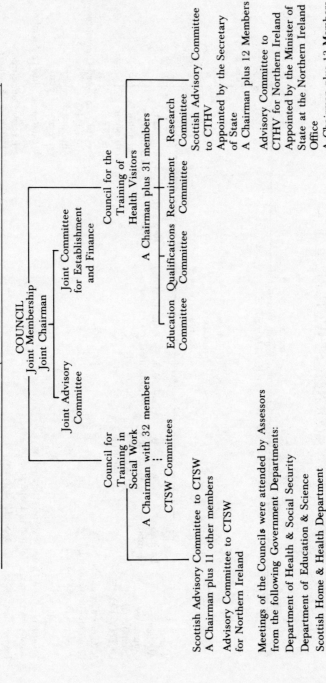

COUNCIL
Joint Membership
Joint Chairman

Joint Advisory Committee

Joint Committee for Establishment and Finance

Council for Training in Social Work
A Chairman with 32 members

CTSW Committees

Scottish Advisory Committee to CTSW
A Chairman plus 11 other members

Advisory Committee to CTSW for Northern Ireland

Council for the Training of Health Visitors
A Chairman plus 31 members

Education Committee

Qualifications Committee

Recruitment Committee

Research Committee

Scottish Advisory Committee to CTHV
Appointed by the Secretary of State
A Chairman plus 12 Members

Advisory Committee to CTHV for Northern Ireland
Appointed by the Minister of State at the Northern Ireland Office
A Chairman plus 13 Members

Meetings of the Councils were attended by Assessors from the following Government Departments:
Department of Health & Social Security
Department of Education & Science
Scottish Home & Health Department
Department of Health & Social Services (Northern Ireland)
Welsh Office

Appendix VII

COUNCIL STRUCTURE 1975

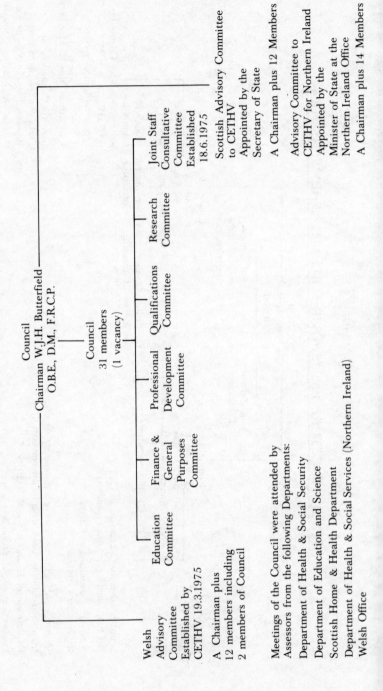

Council
Chairman W.J.H. Butterfield
O.B.E., D.M., F.R.C.P.

Council
31 members
(1 vacancy)

Welsh
Advisory
Committee
Established by
CETHV 19.3.1975

Education
Committee

Finance &
General
Purposes
Committee

Professional
Development
Committee

Qualifications
Committee

Research
Committee

Joint Staff
Consultative
Committee
Established
18.6.1975

Scottish Advisory Committee
to CETHV
Appointed by the
Secretary of State

A Chairman plus 12 Members

Advisory Committee to
CETHV for Northern Ireland
Appointed by the
Minister of State at the
Northern Ireland Office

A Chairman plus 14 Members

A Chairman plus
12 members including
2 members of Council

Meetings of the Council were attended by
Assessors from the following Departments:
Department of Health & Social Security
Department of Education and Science
Scottish Home & Health Department
Department of Health & Social Services (Northern Ireland)
Welsh Office

Appendix VIII

COUNCIL FOR THE EDUCATION AND TRAINING OF HEALTH VISITORS

ADMINISTRATIVE STRUCTURE 1975

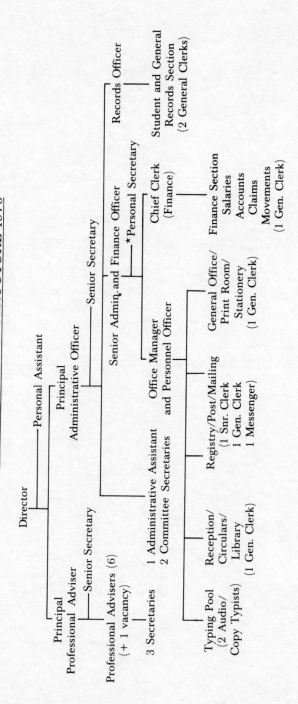

★ Also for Records Officer

Index